*How to understand
and support*
children with
hearing difficulties

Wendy Brown

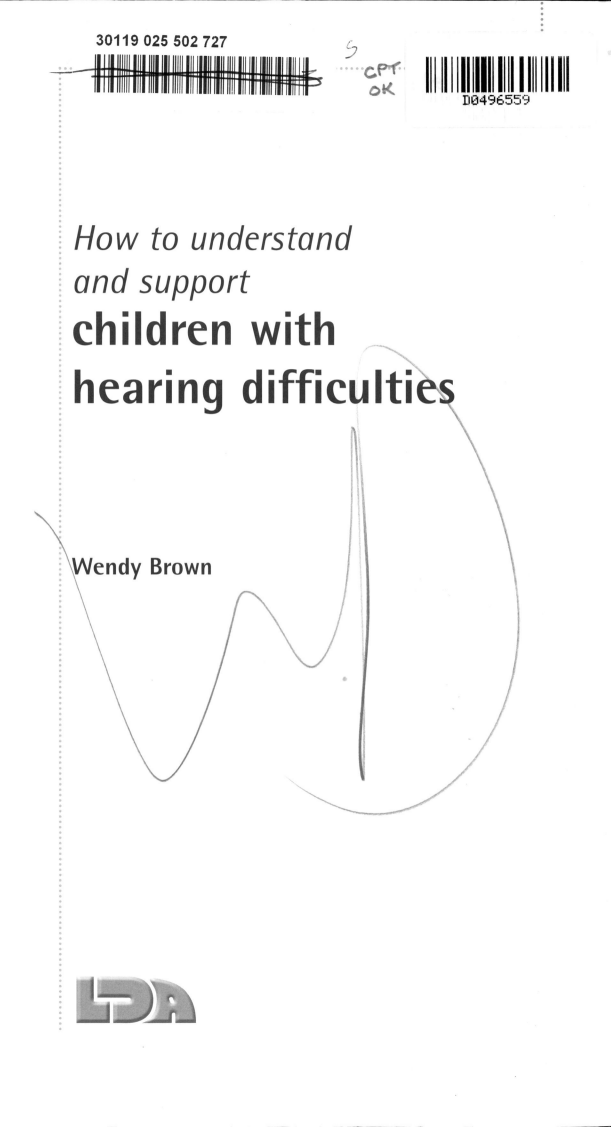

LDA

Acknowledgements

I should like to thank all the many friends and colleagues with whom I have worked over the years, without whom none of this would have been possible.

With thanks to RNID.

Permission to photocopy

This book contains materials which may be reproduced by photocopier or other means for use by the purchaser. This permission is granted on the understanding that these copies will be used within the educational establishment of the purchaser. This book and all its contents remain copyright. Copies may be made without reference to the publisher or to the licensing scheme for the making of photocopies operated by the Publishers' Licensing Agency.

The right of Wendy Brown to be identified as author of this work has been asserted by her in accordance with sections 77 and 78 of the Copyright, Designs and Patents Act 1988.

Whilst the advice and information contained in *How to understand and support children with hearing difficulties* are believed to be true and accurate at the time of going to press, RNID nor the author can accept any legal responsibility or liability for any errors or omissions that may be made.

How to understand and support children with hearing difficulties
MT10001
ISBN-13: 978 1 85503 402 0

© Wendy Brown
Cover illustration © Rebecca Barnes
Inside illustrations © Rebecca Barnes
All rights reserved
First published 2006
Reprinted 2007

Printed in the UK for LDA
Abbeygate House, East Road, Cambridge, CB1 1DB, UK

Contents

Contents

Introduction

Who is this book for?

The information in this book will provide a valuable resource for the full range of school staff coming into contact with children experiencing temporary or permanent hearing difficulties. It is written to appeal to those who have little or no previous experience of this very special group and aims to provide clear guidelines for all concerned. Parents will find it provides a valuable insight into the systems and approaches supporting their children.

The book outlines causes, types and degrees of deafness and their likely impact on learning styles and needs. Guidance and suggestions on delivery and presentation are provided throughout, along with practical strategies for effective communication and understanding. This book should have particular appeal to adults involved with Key Stages 1 and 2, but the information is relevant to staff working at all stages and in all types of provision.

What are the educational implications of a hearing loss?

A school is first and foremost a listening environment:

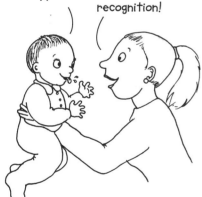

Blurble, blurble, thrupphh!

You're so right, darling! There is a link between phonic awareness and language recognition!

- We copy what we hear. If a child cannot detect the human voice clearly, their own speech is unlikely to be clear. Babies 'burble' instinctively, and this is reinforced by the satisfaction of hearing their own voices and getting positive responses from others. As they mature, their utterances become recognisable and their words meaningful as they copy what they hear other people saying. If a child cannot hear clearly enough to discriminate between sounds and cannot hear phonetic distinctions in the first 12 months of life, they are likely to experience significant language learning problems.

- Reading is a skill based on language acquisition. Therefore, a deaf child may have delayed literacy development.

- A delay in acquiring literacy skills may have an impact on all aspects of a child's access to the curriculum, and on their self-esteem and confidence.

- Classroom management is important. A child with a hearing loss needs to be near the main speaker. Contributions from other class members should be repeated so that the deaf child understands how the topic is developing.

- Children with hearing difficulties may not overhear discussions. They may need to be taught concepts, vocabulary and social clues on a organised and structured basis. Other children will often learn these things incidentally.

- Children experiencing difficulties in acquiring language through listening may struggle to develop the ability to think or express themselves abstractly. Difficulties include concepts of time, emotions and use of synonyms.

- Social integration is affected by a lack of speech and language. Feelings of isolation and confusion can interrupt learning.

- Individuals whose deafness dates from early life have increased vulnerability to emotional and mental health problems.

There have been positive developments in relation to the child with hearing difficulties in the mainstream classroom. The identification, intervention and support available for deaf children is far better than it used to be and continues to improve. More children are now expected to have age-appropriate attainments. Due to the roll-out of newborn hearing screening, resulting in the prescription of digital hearing aids for very young babies and the fitting of cochlear implants at around a year old, children have access to sound and language from a much earlier age. In addition, there is greater support from teachers of the deaf (ToDs) to families from the time of diagnosis, and more extensive in-school support and advice as children grow older. This has a direct impact on children's educational and social achievements, and ensures that teaching a deaf child will be a rewarding and enriching experience.

The trend towards inclusion of deaf children

There has been a slow but steady policy of educating children with hearing difficulties in mainstream schools since the first resource base attached to one was opened in the 1960s. Gradually, legislation plus technological advances in audiological provision have made inclusion more viable and desirable.

Children with hearing difficulties are increasingly benefiting from higher expectations, increased levels of appropriate and targeted support, and greater access to opportunities. School staff are acquiring the knowledge, understanding and ability to extend their professional skills. Whole school communities are enriched by the inclusion and acceptance of diversity.

Developing whole-school strategies

At the heart of any inclusion policy is the concept of equality of opportunity.

All schools lay claim to a commitment to equality of opportunity in all aspects of school life. However, the recent focus on league tables, testing and developing strategies for accessing the academic curriculum has sometimes meant that we have taken our eye off the hidden curriculum. The following points of discussion will help you to examine the situation in your school:

- ❍ Putting the National Curriculum to one side, what else do children learn in school? Who teaches them this?
- ❍ What opportunities should be available for all children?
- ❍ How is a positive attitude to special needs issues demonstrated?
- ❍ Does the school recognise discrimination?
- ❍ How does the school deal with aspects of discrimination?

Some of the areas that should be considered when evaluating the relevance of any policy on whole-school strategies are identified in this list:
① When the school is considering new buildings and refurbishment, are the needs of the deaf children made explicit to the architects and designers? Although legislation is in place to ensure that consideration is given to some needs, this is often lost along the way. Who is keeping an eye on this? Do

they know what is best? For example, in Canada and the United States, new schools for the deaf are often built with corridors without corners. Why would that be advantageous for a child with a hearing difficulty?

② Are the resources in the library appropriate for deaf learners, and is the spending reflecting their needs? What about British Sign Language (BSL) online dictionaries, for example?

③ Does the school subscribe to relevant specialist journals?

④ Do the school resources reflect an awareness of deafness? If you pin up information posters, is that enough? Are deaf children mentioned in your reading schemes? Are the displays inclusive? Are deaf adults part of the actual or virtual environment?

⑤ Are technical aids in evidence in all areas of the school or only in the classroom? What facilities does the school office have if a deaf child needs to contact home or if the school needs to contact a deaf parent? Are the fire alarms useful only to the hearing?

⑥ Is the school aware of what is available to ensure equality? Do they know where to look? Do they understand inequality in all its forms?

⑦ Are visiting speakers made aware that they may be expected to use a radio transmitter in assembly or class? Who prepares them?

⑧ Do the plans made for trips out of school include questions about the needs that a deaf child has in a different environment? Who asks the questions? Who has the answers?

This book touches only lightly on some of the issues involved in inclusion. All schools know the benefits that follow self-evaluation.

Informing other children

The successful integration of a child with a hearing difficulty into the mainstream classroom involves the children as much as the adults. They need preparation and information to help them in this situation. Young children will ask straightforward yet penetrating questions, and it is wise to be prepared with clear, unambiguous and informative answers. It would perhaps be helpful to provide a short deaf awareness course. You could ask someone with understanding and experience of deaf issues in education to help you.

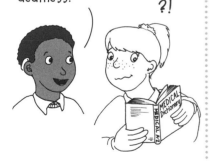

You asked why I can't hear. I have genetic damage to the hair cells in my cochlea, leading to sensori-neural deafness.

?!

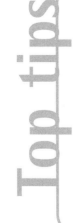

Top tips

- Explain the facts in a non-emotional, non-judgemental manner.
- Try to answer all questions, and tell the class if you do not know something. Find out and tell them at a later date.
- Tell the deaf child in advance if you are planning to teach about hearing difficulties. It would also be advisable to prepare a deaf child in advance if teaching about sound in the science curriculum.
- Don't assume that the deaf child is an expert on all aspects of hearing loss and subsequent difficulties. Although it is natural to want to include a deaf child in any explanations, they should not be required to demonstrate any of their difficulties in order to make a teaching point. Highlighting their strengths will be a far more effective course of action. You should be sensitive to the potential for embarrassment and/or distress.

Top tips

- Don't avoid issues because they present a challenging situation. Seek help from those with experience. If you demonstrate avoidance and lack of knowledge, this may be interpreted by children as a negative attitude and they may copy it.
- Demonstrating a positive attitude is as much about the way we behave as what we say. If you don't have a visible routine for checking hearing aids, the children will not appreciate their value or purpose. (You will find out about these systems later.)
- Allow children to look at and handle hearing aids, but treat them as you would other personal belongings. Spare hearing aids can be borrowed for demonstration, as can ear moulds. Do not allow a child's own hearing aid to be handled.
- There are plenty of resources and training packages available on DVD or video, where explanations are presented in a familiar and entertaining way.
- Don't be tempted to teach fingerspelling and basic signing skills at the expense of other communication tactics. Children enjoy learning sign language, but they also need to know about empathy, lip reading, body language, eye contact and so on.
- Demonstrate the message of inclusion in all you do.

The girls I like best are a bit naughty so I'm not allowed to sit with them.

Louise, aged 6

Attainment and achievement

Since the 1990s there has been emphasis on measuring and recording children's attainment in school through the standardised tests of SATs and GCSEs. Deaf children are making excellent and well-deserved progress alongside their hearing peers in both core and foundation subjects, as evidenced in the statistics available through the Department for Education and Skills (DfES), examination boards and local education authorities (LEAs).

There has been a huge amount of research into the achievements of deaf children and into less easily assessed areas such as communication skills, use of amplification, types and levels of support, self-esteem, friendship, career paths and so on. Information is available from the organisations listed under *Useful contacts* (see page 64).

Audiological equipment

This book provides a considerable amount of information about the audiological equipment in daily use in classrooms. Adults coming into contact with children using this equipment must understand and feel confident about handling and using it.

Terminology

All specialist areas have their own language and vocabulary, which assists greatly in discussion and shared understanding. A glossary of terms is provided to help readers (see page 62). The terms 'hearing difficulties' and 'deaf' are used in the text to relate to a child with an educationally significant hearing loss (greater than an average of 40dB in the better ear).

Chapter 1
What are hearing difficulties?

Hearing in school

Everything done in school depends to some extent on a child's ability to hear well. Any child who experiences difficulty in hearing the voices of adults and children will be disadvantaged and their development affected. In order to understand and support these children, it helps to have a basic awareness of the function, structure and mechanics of the human ear. There are three major functions of hearing.

- ◗ At a primitive level – there are many sounds in the background that help us to identify where we are. The sounds in the home are different from those in school. Our bodies make noises all the time, such as those of breathing and swallowing.

- ◗ At a signal warning level – we use our hearing constantly to monitor the environment. Understanding what is happening around us when we cannot see events gives us security.

- ◗ At a spoken communication level – although the human ear responds to a great variety of environmental noise, it is at its most sensitive when responding to the sound of the human voice. Speech develops naturally because we learn to listen, process, copy and practise. There is a huge incentive to succeed as we are continually rewarded by increasingly complex interactions with others. We also learn that with good communication strategies we can determine the outcomes of situations.

Structure of the human ear

There are three major parts to the ear. The outer ear consists of:

- ◗ the auricle (also called the pinna) – the visible part of the outer ear;
- ◗ the ear canal – a tubular passage that runs from the pinna to the ear drum;
- ◗ the ear drum (tympanic membrane) – the membrane that closes the inner end of the ear canal and moves in response to sound waves.

The middle ear is an air-filled cavity – an area set in the bones of the skull and about the size of a small sugar cube. It contains:

- ◗ the ossicles – three small bones connecting the ear drum to the oval window of the inner ear, called the malleus, incus and stapes (commonly known as the hammer, anvil and stirrup);
- ◗ the Eustachian tube – a passage linking the nasal cavity and the middle ear cavity, which helps to balance the air pressure in the middle ear and to drain the chamber of any gathering fluid or mucus.

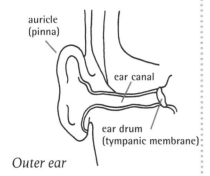

Outer ear

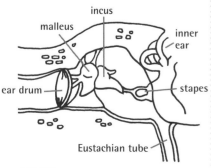

Middle ear

The inner ear consists of:

○ the oval window – the entrance to the fluid-filled cavity of the inner ear;

○ the cochlea – a shell-shaped structure containing sensory hair cells, lying deep in the temporal bones of the skull;

○ three semi-circular canals – the organs of balance;

○ the auditory nerve – which takes neural signals from the cochlea to the brain.

How does the ear work?

Air particles are set into vibration by a physical disturbance to form travelling sound waves. The sound waves are collected by the pinna and funnelled down the ear canal towards the ear drum. The movement of the condensed sound waves is transmitted to the tautly stretched ear drum to make it vibrate. The vibration continues to carry the sound through the three middle-ear bones to the inner ear. The waves arrive at the oval window in the form of amplified mechanical energy. The force exerted by the stirrup on the oval window of the cochlea is converted into hydraulic pressure waves. The waves pass swiftly through the fluid-filled inner ear, stimulating thousands of sensory hair cells, which produce small electrical charges. The electrical signals travel along the auditory nerve and through enormously complex neural pathways to the brain. The brain recognises, analyses and interprets the signals.

General causes of hearing loss

Hearing difficulties in children may be due to a wide variety of conditions occurring in any part of the ear at any time in the child's development. During pregnancy and around the time of birth a number of potentially hazardous events may occur, some associated with subsequent hearing loss. In early life the child is exposed to a variety of influences which may impair hearing. These fall into three groups:

○ *Pre-natal* – rubella, viruses and infections. These may be contracted by the mother during pregnancy.

○ *Peri-natal* – prematurity, difficulties with breathing soon after birth (resulting in oxygen deficiency), severe jaundice, prolonged or difficult labour, rhesus incompatibility.

○ *Post-natal* – secretory otitis media, childhood fevers (e.g. mumps and measles), meningitis, head injury, ototoxic drugs, exposure to loud noise, tumours on auditory nerve.

Genetic causes of hearing loss

The genetically determined conditions associated with deafness include Down syndrome, Treacher Collins syndrome, cleft lip and palate, and Usher syndrome. They are relatively uncommon and beyond the scope of this book. The support services for these conditions will provide guidance.

Tinnitus

Tinnitus may be generated in the ears, the nerves associated with hearing, or the auditory pathways to the brain. It may be perceived as ringing, humming,

View of ear from front

middle ear space

ear canal

cochlea

Eustachian tube

Secretory otitis media: One in five young children at any one time may suffer from this condition, often known as Glue Ear (see page 17).

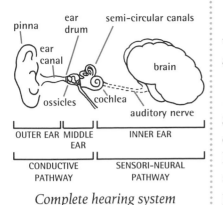

Complete hearing system

whistling or some other type or combination of sound. Often associated with ageing, it may affect people of all ages. Sufferers may or may not be deaf.

Non-organic loss

Some children appear to be experiencing hearing difficulties when in fact they do not have a significant loss. There is no organic cause for their apparent hearing problems. They often demonstrate over-reliance on lip reading and say they cannot hear. This may be a symptom of an underlying psychological problem, or an auditory processing disorder (APD).

Causes of different types of hearing loss

Outer ear	Middle ear	Inner ear
Impacted wax in ear canal	Middle-ear infections	Noise exposure
Foreign objects in ear canal	Congenital conditions	Congenital conditions
Damage to ear drum	Otosclerosis	Ototoxic drugs
Atresia or stenosis	Damage to ossicles	Environmental causes
		Prematurity
		Pre-, peri- and post-natal complications

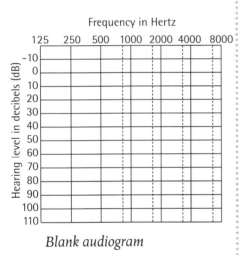

Blank audiogram

Types of hearing loss

- If either the outer or middle ear is not working properly, the hearing loss is known as a *conductive* loss. This may be temporary.
- Damage to the inner ear results in *sensori-neural* hearing loss. This is generally a permanent condition.
- A mixed loss occurs when there is a problem in both middle and inner ear.

How do we measure and describe hearing loss?

It is important to understand:

- how hearing is measured;
- how hearing loss is described and the terminology used by professionals;
- how to read an audiogram;
- how to discuss the child's hearing loss in an informed way.

Hearing can be tested with a machine called an audiometer. The results are recorded on a chart known as an audiogram, which is in the form of a graph. The horizontal axis measures frequency (pitch) in Hertz (Hz). In a hearing test the audiologist usually tests at 250, 500, 1000, 2000, 4000 and 8000Hz. The higher the number, the higher the frequency (pitch) of the sound. The vertical axis measures the loudness of sounds in decibels (dB).

The audiologist tests each frequency at different loudness levels, starting with loud sounds that are easy to hear. The audiometer can make sounds up to 110dB, which is very loud. Gradually the sounds become softer until they are difficult to hear. The quietest level that can be heard for each frequency is called the threshold. The audiologist marks the graph to indicate the threshold.

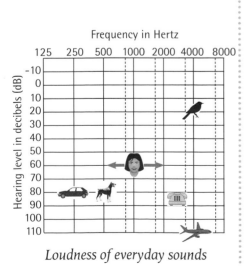

Loudness of everyday sounds

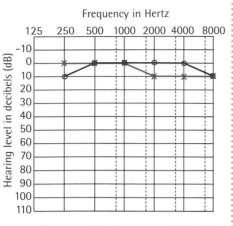

Audiogram showing normal hearing

Each ear is tested and plotted separately, using a red circle for right and a blue cross for left. People normally have thresholds of 0–20dB. All of their Os and Xs are near the top of the audiogram. If a child has a hearing loss, the Xs and Os will not be near the top of the audiogram. A child may not hear a frequency until it is much louder than 0dB. If they can hear a frequency only at 50dB or louder, their threshold is 50dB at that frequency.

The frequencies of 500, 1000 and 2000 are those of almost all speech sounds. A child who has trouble hearing them will have difficulty hearing speech sounds. The shaded 'speech banana' on the audiograms below indicates where normal conversational speech occurs. The further down the graph the Xs and Os are plotted, the greater the hearing loss. If hearing aids are prescribed, the child's hearing will be retested to establish their thresholds whilst wearing the aids.

It is quite common for the hearing in each ear to be different:
- ◐ Deafness in both ears is described as *bilateral*.
- ◐ Deafness in one ear is described as *unilateral*.
- ◐ A similar loss in both ears is described as *symmetrical*.
- ◐ A different loss in each ear is described as *asymmetrical*.

The results are also described by the shape on the completed audiogram: flat, sloping, ski slope, or left-hand corner.

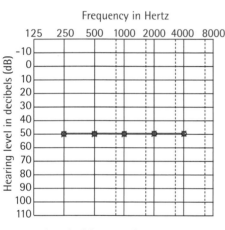

Thresholds of 50dB in both ears

The degree of hearing loss is calculated on an average based on five different frequencies in the better ear:
- ◐ Mild = 21–40dB average loss in the better ear.
- ◐ Moderate = 41–70dB average loss in the better ear.
- ◐ Severe = 71–95dB average loss in the better ear.
- ◐ Profound = in excess of 95dB average loss in the better ear.

A comprehensive description of an individual child's hearing loss should include: the degree, the type and shape, whether both ears are affected, the age of onset and further appropriate comments (e.g. progressive, fluctuating).

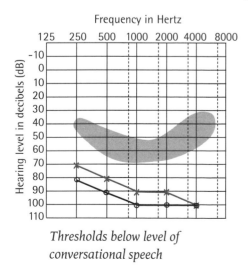

Thresholds below level of conversational speech

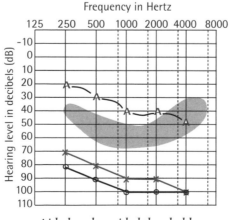

Aided and unaided thresholds

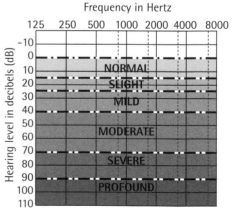

Degree of hearing loss

Chapter 2
Identifying children with hearing loss

Hearing difficulties can arise at any time and for a variety of reasons. Be on the lookout for children who appear to be experiencing some difficulty in hearing. Children with conductive, mixed and sensori-neural loss may go undetected. Checklist 1 will help you to identify hearing problems.

What to do next

Don't immediately assume that lots of ticks in the Yes column of Checklist 1 mean the child is deaf. Take the following action:

- Check the pupil's records.
- Ask the parents if the child has any history of hearing loss.
- Check the referral procedures in your LEA. The local special needs advisory services should have given you the information you need. If not, ask them.
- You can usually refer to the school nurse, who will do a sweep test. This is a routine test carried out on entry to school in most parts of the UK. It checks if the child can hear four frequencies at a set dB level. If necessary, the school nurse will refer the child to an audiologist.
- Suggest the parents take the child to their GP.

Checklist 2 may be useful to collect information for a specific child.

Checklist 3 presents the suggested referral procedure diagrammatically. The child may have a learning difficulty other than one concerned with hearing. It is easy to overlook warning signs when concentrating on another medical condition or obstacle to learning. Multi-agency involvement may be necessary initially, but some services will not get involved until hearing loss has been ruled out as a reason for difficulties in learning.

After diagnosis

If after diagnosis you don't have a clear explanation for the child's condition, contact your local advisory service for more information. You could ask the parents to tell you where the child was tested, and contact the audiologist involved for a detailed explanation and prognosis.

The referral process may take a considerable time. While you are waiting, you can adopt some of the advice in Chapter 3. Even if hearing loss is not diagnosed, this may prove helpful. In cases where a moderate or severe hearing loss is diagnosed and the child is prescribed a hearing aid, you should be contacted by a ToD, who will provide basic Inset training. If you already have a ToD regularly visiting your school, you can ask them for help, information and guidance.

It is estimated that one in four children will suffer a temporary hearing loss at some time, usually between the age of 4 and 8.

Checklist 1 – Signs of possible hearing loss

Name of child _____

	Yes	No
Section 1 – Physical signs		
Frequent earache or infections/catarrh	☐	☐
Discharge from ears	☐	☐
Frequent upper-respiratory-tract infections	☐	☐
Frequently rubs ears	☐	☐
Frequently breathes with mouth open	☐	☐
Section 2 – Receptive signs		
Delay in response to instructions compared to majority of peers	☐	☐
Mislocates sound source	☐	☐
Misunderstanding or confusion of verbal instructions	☐	☐
Strains to listen	☐	☐
Turns head to one side when listening	☐	☐
Fails to respond if addressed from behind or from a reasonable distance	☐	☐
Gets close to speaker	☐	☐
Watches speaker's face and lips intently	☐	☐
Relies on following other children when starting and stopping an activity	☐	☐
Requires speaker to raise voice	☐	☐
Responds less well in large room (e.g. dining hall, hall)	☐	☐
Seems to hear, then not hear (e.g. responds to own name at a distance, but not to simple commands at same distance)	☐	☐
Inattentive for no obvious reason	☐	☐

Signs of possible hearing loss

Section 3 – Expressive signs	Yes	No
Frequently asks for things to be repeated	☐	☐
Frequently says *Eh?, What?, Pardon*	☐	☐
Misanswers questions	☐	☐
Immature or indistinct speech	☐	☐
Nasal-sounding speech	☐	☐
Unusually loud or quiet voice	☐	☐
Difficulty learning to say new words	☐	☐
Significantly poorer vocabulary than school peers	☐	☐
Nodding or smiling, then doing wrong thing	☐	☐
Asking questions about something already or recently explained	☐	☐
Slow progress in learning to read	☐	☐
Erratic educational performance	☐	☐

Section 4 – Social/behavioural signs		
Loses concentration	☐	☐
Shows signs of frustration/anxiety/stress/aggression	☐	☐
Difficulty in making social relationships	☐	☐
Tires easily	☐	☐
Clumsy	☐	☐
Reluctant to attend school	☐	☐
Parents/guardian express concern about child's hearing	☐	☐

Other concerns or comments _____

_____

_____

_____

_____

SENCo: _____

Class teacher: _____

Date: _____

Checklist 2 – Suspected hearing impairment

Name of child: _____   Date of birth: _____

School: _____   Home address: _____

School records checked for evidence of hearing impairment   Date: _____

Findings: _____
_____
_____
_____

Name of consultant: _____

Hospital involved: _____

Referred to (school nurse / GP / audiologist):   Date: _____
_____

Findings: _____
_____
_____

Unresolved concerns about this child: _____
_____
_____

Parents/guardian of child informed   Date: _____

Referred to: _____   Date: _____

Outline of parents' concerns: _____
_____
_____

Is the child on the Code of Practice Register?   Yes ☐ No ☐

If 'Yes', circle below as appropriate and provide brief details.

School Action   School Action Plus   Under assessment for Statement   Statement

Outline reasons: _____
_____
_____

What is Glue Ear?

Glue Ear (otitis media) is a form of temporary conductive hearing loss and the most common cause of hearing problems in childhood. This section focuses on the background to the condition and how to help those affected by it.

Glue Ear represents a serious developmental hazard to children even after it has been treated and far more children suffer from undiagnosed Glue Ear than hitherto thought.

Dr Alec Webster (1988), 'Conditions: glue ear', *Special Children*, 20

Glue Ear affects the mechanism of the middle ear. The ear drum is stretched over the entrance to the middle ear. Condensed sound waves are transmitted to the drum, which moves in and out. This vibration continues to be transmitted through the middle-ear bones (ossicles) to the inner ear. The vibration arrives at the entrance to the inner ear in the form of amplified energy. The Eustachian tube must open and close to keep the air pressure on each side of the ear drum equal. In children this tube is not as straight and wide as when they are older, and does not always work well. If it cannot open, the air in the middle-ear cavity is absorbed into the surrounding tissues and the ear drum is sucked inwards and becomes tighter. It is then unable to vibrate freely in response to sound waves. If the Eustachian tube remains blocked, a watery fluid is produced in the middle-ear space. This makes it difficult for the ossicles to move and pass the sound signals to the inner ear. Fluid within the middle ear can cause intermittent problems with hearing. This is very confusing for the child and for adults living and working with them. The fluid may thicken to a glue-like consistency (Glue Ear).

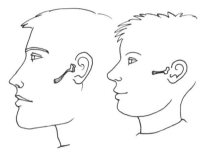

Difference between child and adult Eustachian tube

How is hearing affected?

It becomes harder for sound to be conducted, so sounds are missed or distorted. The effect is like listening with both fingers stuck into your ears. Bone is a conductor of sound. A child with Glue Ear may be responding to vibration transmitted through the bones of the skull. This is not an efficient way of conducting sound, and it adds to the erratic nature of the child's responses to sound.

Almost twice as many boys as girls suffer from a temporary conductive loss.

Factors that contribute to the development of Glue Ear include repeated colds and flu, and passive smoking. Children with genetic conditions such as Down syndrome are susceptible as they may have smaller Eustachian tubes and produce thicker mucus. If you are concerned that a child may be experiencing fluctuating hearing loss, use Checklist 1 (pages 14–15) to help you identify the problem.

Treatment

In the vast majority of cases, the condition improves after a course of antibiotics or decongestants. If it persists, surgical treatment may be necessary, involving the removal of the adenoids and/or tonsils.

Surgery to insert a grommet is sometimes necessary. The grommet is a very small plastic tube which acts as a substitute for the Eustachian tube and helps to diminish the amount of fluid. The ear drums are punctured and the fluid is aspirated using a suction tube. A grommet is inserted through the opening in the ear drum. Most grommets are designed to come out on their own, working

Checklist 3 – Typical referral procedures

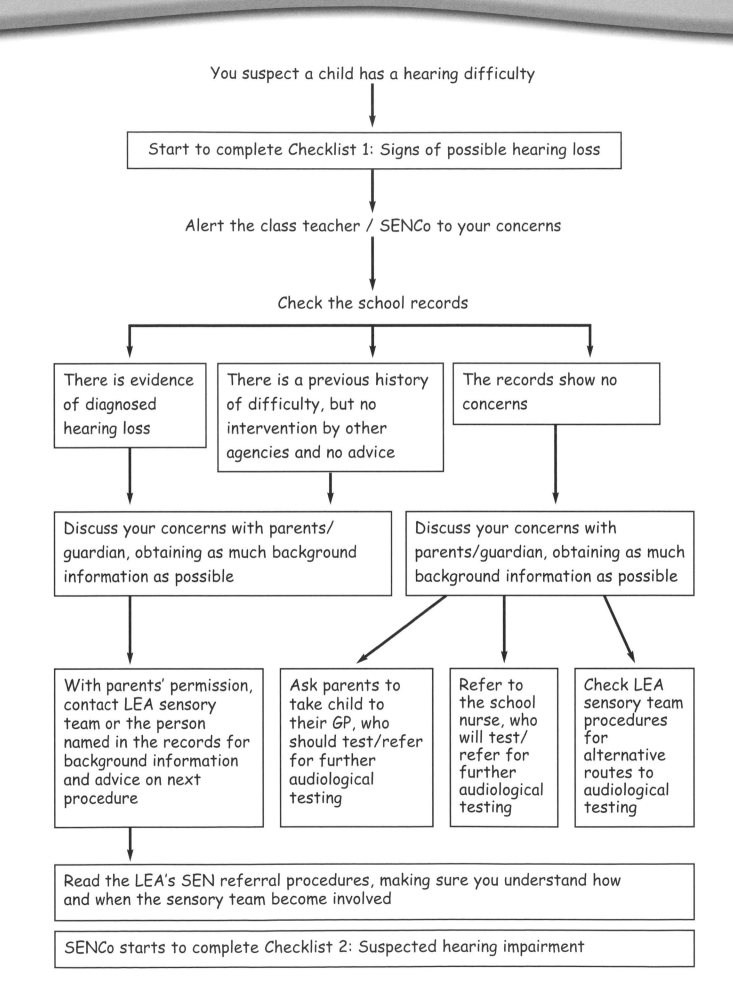

You suspect a child has a hearing difficulty

Start to complete Checklist 1: Signs of possible hearing loss

Alert the class teacher / SENCo to your concerns

Check the school records

| There is evidence of diagnosed hearing loss | There is a previous history of difficulty, but no intervention by other agencies and no advice | The records show no concerns |

Discuss your concerns with parents/guardian, obtaining as much background information as possible

Discuss your concerns with parents/guardian, obtaining as much background information as possible

With parents' permission, contact LEA sensory team or the person named in the records for background information and advice on next procedure

Ask parents to take child to their GP, who should test/refer for further audiological testing

Refer to the school nurse, who will test/refer for further audiological testing

Check LEA sensory team procedures for alternative routes to audiological testing

Read the LEA's SEN referral procedures, making sure you understand how and when the sensory team become involved

SENCo starts to complete Checklist 2: Suspected hearing impairment

Insertion of a grommet into the ear drum

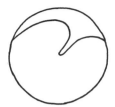

1. Ear drum

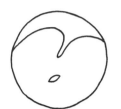

2. Small opening in ear drum to remove fluid and to insert grommet

3. 'Shah' grommet

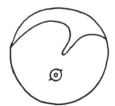

4. Grommet in ear drum

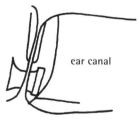

ear canal

5. Grommet tube seen in cross-section

their way out with wax. They sometimes fall out prematurely, and they may become blocked, affecting hearing.

Children fitted with grommets may go in water with ear protection. They should not swim under water or dive.

Practical classroom strategies

Following an operation for the insertion of grommets, the hearing mechanism starts to work normally again, but it would be unwise to assume that the child's functional hearing has been restored immediately. Like children with Glue Ear who have repeated bouts of conductive hearing loss but have not had surgery, they need special attention. Children who have experienced reduced and inconsistent auditory input over a long period may have not understood or even heard some of the key elements of speech and language. This may need remediation and constant monitoring. Hearing aids are not normally offered to children with Glue Ear. However, Sound Field Systems (SFS) have been shown to help. See Chapter 4 for more information.

How to help these children in the mainstream classroom:

- Seat the child near the front and slightly to one side. This gives them a clear view of you and also enables them to follow classmates' contributions.
- Get the child's attention before you start talking and before changing topic.
- Face the child as much as possible, using eye contact and speaking clearly.
- Keep background noise to a minimum. Listening conditions are important as incidental noise can be disproportionately confusing.
- Regularly check their understanding.
- Include them in group discussion.
- Maintain your normal pace and rhythm of speech.
- Avoid shouting or mouthing artificially.
- Ensure that the child is aware of who is speaking. Use the names of children before accepting their contribution to enable the deaf child to face the speaker. This takes practice as it involves a slight adjustment of pace. Alternatively, repeat all contributions so everyone receives the information.

Long-term impact of fluctuating hearing loss

All children need consistent auditory input for optimum linguistic development, and the effect of even a mild fluctuating loss should not be underestimated. It will have a particularly significant impact on children who are already demonstrating difficulties in learning. Children with reading difficulties, behaviour problems, poor attention skills, speech and language difficulties, and poor achievement are all vulnerable to long-term effects.

Young children do not have the linguistic or auditory experience to predict the content of what is being said to them, so they cannot compensate for the distorted stimuli they receive when they have a conductive hearing loss. The child will make inaccurate decisions which impede language coding, because they lack the strategies to cope with the same input in different acoustic formats. For example, *cats* could be heard as *ca*, *at* or *a*, and the child may not realise that they are the same word. The child may demonstrate subsequent communication difficulties.

Receptive language

The child's ability to discriminate high-frequency speech sounds such as voiceless fricatives *s*, *sh*, *f*, *t* and *d* may have been affected by alterations in early auditory input. The child would have missed the consonants that mark tense, possession and number. These also occur in important function words.

In spoken language, turn taking is dependent on the detection of the prosodic features of speech. The child may misunderstand speech sounds and the prosodic message of language.

Auditory discrimination

In a noisy classroom the child may have difficulty in locating a sound quickly. This will prevent them from listening to the appropriate speaker. Background sounds such as noise from the corridors or outside windows may mask speech.

Semantics

Initial vocabulary development may be slower, but should follow normal patterns if appropriate stimulation is given. There may be some auditory confusions, such as between *mouth* and *mouse*.

Expressive language

The child may use more simple syntax in sentences than others of similar age and may demonstrate problems with markers at the end of words (*-s*, *-ed*, *-n't*, *-s* and *-est*), which reflect comprehension difficulties caused by the hearing loss. They may demonstrate errors of agreement between subject and verb.

Speech

There may be problems with phonology (segmental) and, to a lesser degree, with prosody (suprasegmental). The child may omit the final consonants in words, be confused by voice/voiceless sounds (e.g. *t/d*) and cluster reduction (e.g. *sk* becomes *k* and *sky* becomes *ky*).

General manifestations

The child will:

- have difficulty in discriminating the teacher's voice against classroom noise;
- have difficulty when spoken to from behind;
- become tired easily because of the need to put extra effort into listening;
- probably have difficulty in concentrating for any length of time.

Chapter 3
Meeting the needs of children with hearing loss

I didn't understand why the others seemed to know what to do straightaway.

Sarah, aged 7

This chapter looks at the different problems encountered by children with specific losses and how you might start to address their particular needs. Children with fluctuating conductive loss are discussed in Chapter 2.

Children with mild hearing loss

Children with this type of loss often:

- are upset in a noisy classroom and obviously struggle to hear;
- are inattentive and respond more slowly than expected;
- appear to hear in some situations and not others;
- have difficulty in locating sound and may turn in the wrong direction;
- behave as though they haven't heard or understood an instruction.

How to help

- Try to place the child near the teacher.
- Make sure that the child can see the rest of the class and is not sitting with their back to most of the action. They will rely on cues from others if they have not understood or heard you properly.
- Try to get the child's attention when you are speaking to their group or the whole class. Saying the child's name before you start is often sufficient.
- Do not become irritated if the child repeatedly misunderstands. They will already be aware that others understand or hear more easily than they can.

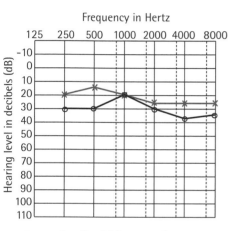

Example of mild hearing loss

Children with unilateral loss

Children with this type of loss often:

- ask for repetition;
- detect sound but may have trouble locating it;
- become confused when more than one person is talking;
- appear confused when there is background noise;
- are reluctant to join in group discussion;
- have delayed reading ability;
- have difficulties in hearing on the sports field or in the playground;
- are tired and irritable.

How to help

- Establish which is the child's better ear and seat them to the best advantage. As a general rule, the better ear should be directed towards the source of the

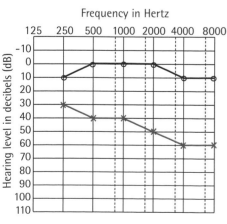

Example of unilateral loss

teacher's voice. The worse ear should face the source of unwanted noise such as passing traffic, open windows, corridors and open doors.

- Encourage other pupils to speak clearly.
- Repeat instructions and explanations; use the board to list key points and new vocabulary.
- Endeavour to create a good listening environment. (There is more about this in Chapters 4 and 5.) Keep classroom noise to a minimum.
- Make sure the pupil can see you.

Children with high-frequency loss

Children with this type of loss often:

- can detect speech but have difficulties with speech discernability (i.e. it is audible but not intelligible);
- have 'slushy' speech themselves, which indicates that they may be having trouble hearing high-frequency consonant sounds like s and sh;
- have difficulty incorporating phonics into their literacy development;
- cannot hear other pupils' contributions in class;
- misunderstand situations owing to mishearing what other people say;
- produce written work that omits word endings, plurals and words they have difficulty hearing;
- have speech with unusual patterns of intonation.

How to help

- Seat the child so they have a good view of the room. If they need to turn round to 'watch' an answer, make sure you either use the name of the child answering or point to them so that the child knows where to look. Repeating the answer, right or wrong, will reduce misunderstandings.
- Try to keep reasonably still. It is very hard for a child to watch a face that is continually moving around the room. That may also attract unwelcome attention to the deaf child, who may be the only one actually looking at you.
- Familiarise yourself with the child's hearing aid if one has been prescribed. If you feel confident that you understand what it can and cannot do, you can help the child make the best use of it. (See Chapter 4 for more about this.)
- Pay attention to lighting. Don't stand in front of windows or bright lights.
- Remember that raising your voice distorts the sound.
- If a child cannot hear a phrase clearly, repeating it verbatim may not help at all. Rephrasing it or changing the word order may help, for example:

Where have you left the atlas?
Change to
The atlas, do you know where it is?

- Remind children of word endings and plurals throughout tasks.
- Lip reading is exhausting and imprecise, and a child can only lip read a word they know. If introducing new vocabulary to the child, it will take repeated

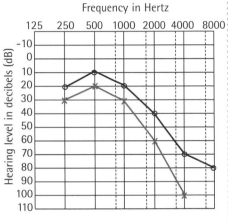

Frequency in Hertz

Example of high-frequency loss

I have to watch the teacher's face all the time. Most of the others are looking out of the window. The teacher thinks I'm a swot. I get asked for most of the answers. It's not fair.

Andrew, aged 11

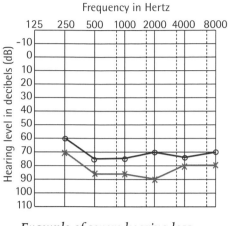

Example of severe hearing loss

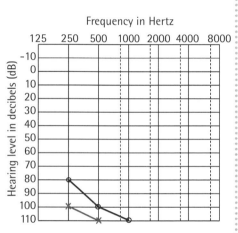

Example of profound hearing loss

Record all or part of one of your lessons. Play it back and ask yourself some searching questions about your delivery, clarity, pace, intelligibility and distractibility.

exposure to match your lips with a known word, phrase or sound. Be patient. Reinforce new vocabulary by writing it on the board.

Children with severe and profound hearing loss

The features presented by children with severe and profound losses are complex, and yet in many ways they are more straightforward than those looked at earlier. Children with this type of loss may:

- need amplification to hear speech;
- not necessarily be able to hear clearly, even with the best amplification available;
- have delayed speech and language skills;
- have delayed literacy skills;
- have substantial gaps in general knowledge;
- have substantial gaps in social skills;
- need considerable 1:1 input;
- need more reinforcement and repetition than a child with normal hearing;
- be more reliant on lip reading;
- have had considerable help from early intervention support agencies and substantial input from a ToD following diagnosis, at whatever age.

How to help

Look at the strategies suggested so far. They are all relevant for children with greater levels of hearing loss. For children with severe or profound loss, more consideration needs to be given to implementing strategies, modifications and approaches. It will take time to incorporate these into your normal classroom delivery, but they will benefit all children, whether deaf or not. You will have help and advice from your local special needs advisory service.

Speaking in class

All teachers have an individual style, pace and manner, and all measure success by the positive responses they get. If you speak with care, clearly and at a natural rate, a deaf child will be able to follow you. They may not understand or hear everything you say, but that won't be because of your delivery. Avoid exaggerating your lip patterns; that distorts what you say.

Use short phrases and sentences rather than individual words.

Children cannot concentrate for long, so do not launch into a continuous monologue. Pace your lesson to include discussion and activities. Deaf children will not respond well if you are constantly interrupted or change the topic unexpectedly mid-sentence. If a deaf child has not understood, change word order, vocabulary or emphasis.

Hearing aids

A child with a severe/profound loss will most likely be using hearing aids and/or have a cochlear implant, possibly with a personal FM system (radio aid). The basic theory and rationale of amplification is explained in Chapter 4. Remember the visiting ToD will give you all the help you need.

You will be asked and expected to wear the transmitter part of the personal FM system as your contribution to making the best use of the child's own useful hearing. Initially, remembering to wear this all the time can be difficult. With a young child it will be your responsibility to remember. With an older child you may need to ask, bargain or hunt for it. Ultimately the child will take responsibility for ensuring it is round your neck and working, but teaching them these things takes time.

Becoming noise aware

We had to sit in alphabetical order. The teacher wouldn't discuss it. I sat next to the same rattling radiator for three years of geography. Most of the time I couldn't hear what he was saying.

John, aged 14

Making an audio tape of a typical lesson would be a useful exercise in order to experience the conditions in the classroom as a participant listener rather than as a teacher, occupied with delivery. Are you noise aware?

- ❍ Do you leave the classroom door open, even when children are moving to and fro?
- ❍ Are you aware of the electrical hum produced by lights, fans, computers and OHPs?
- ❍ Do you leave the window open when the lawn is being mowed?
- ❍ Do you take steps to get noisy radiators fixed?
- ❍ Do you insist that children don't drag their chairs?

Listening conditions in classrooms are discussed in Chapter 4.

Staying in view

Children with hearing difficulties like to watch faces for information, and get cues from natural gestures. Positioning the child so they can see you and other children is sometimes difficult, especially with younger children in flexible contexts. Do your best.

Obviously if the classrooms have rows of desks it is easier to position the child; somewhere towards the front and to the side is preferable. The same principle applies in assemblies. Try to keep them close, especially if they are not using a personal FM system. They need to be within 1–1.5 metres to hear you if they are wearing hearing aids or have a cochlear implant.

Lighting

You need to become light aware, too. Ask yourself these questions:

- ❍ Do all the lights work?
- ❍ Do I switch them on or get so involved that I don't notice it's semi-dark?
- ❍ Do I make sure my face is in the light?
- ❍ Do I know where the areas of shadow are?

○ Would I know what to do for a deaf child if we were watching a presentation in the dark (e.g. a film or PowerPoint presentation)?

○ Do I stand in front of the window, putting myself in shadow?

Understanding and managing divided visual attention

We have already explained that children with hearing difficulties are dependent on face watching and reading body language to supplement the auditory input, which may be unclear or incomplete.

If you are working alongside a child at a computer screen, put a mirror in a position where the child can easily switch their gaze from the screen to your face in the mirror to follow your lip patterns.

Lip patterns can be read this way with a little practice. Remember to allow time for the child to switch attention between the screen and mirror. Can you think of any other situations where a mirror would be useful?

If you are reading aloud to the class, asking the class to follow the text in the book in front of them, the deaf child will not be able to do both simultaneously. They can watch you and try to follow, or they can look at the text and try to keep pace – without necessarily knowing where you are up to.

If the children were working on computers and had their backs to you, how could you expect a deaf child to watch you and follow your instructions whilst continuing to watch the screen and do as you say or understand what you were saying?

There are many situations like these in school. Gradually you will develop strategies to deal with most of them. If you have an in-class support worker, the problems are easier to overcome. If you are working alone you have to do some creative thinking.

Some practical strategies

Try to incorporate these strategies gradually over time; they will soon become second nature:

○ Give visual clues when discussing. A picture says a thousand words. Point, touch and indicate what the topic is and what you are talking about.

○ The closer you hold something to your face, the easier it is for the child to scan between or take in both simultaneously.

○ Experienced deaf children use all the visual clues and use peripheral vision to advantage. Build in moments of time for the child to look up and down, here and there, at your face, then at a model (e.g. of a volcano).

○ Indicate changes of topic. If you are still looking at the lava flow while talking about the arrangements for collecting money for the school trip, the child will be justifiably confused. Indicate a change of topic by writing a new title or some key vocabulary on the board.

○ If you give out text with instructions, allow the child time to read it before asking questions or making comments. If you are explaining while the child is trying to read and process the information, they are less likely to succeed immediately.

○ Avoid talking about the contents of a video whilst it is playing. If you must comment, either stop the video to make the observation or talk about it

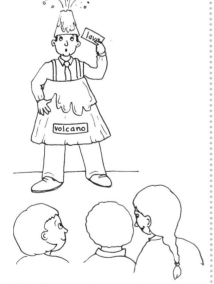

"Mr Benson always puts a lot of effort into making his lessons visual!"

afterwards. Asking the class to look out for specific things before starting is another way to cue the child in.

O Try to use video programmes or DVDs with subtitles. (DVDs often have subtitles as an embedded option. When ordering new DVDs, check whether this feature is available. If not, provide written transcripts to accompany the video.) Subtitles may not be age appropriate and further explanation may be needed. Ideally, the child would be prepared in advance for this.

O Allow the child to borrow the tape to watch again at home, where parents can be involved. Better still, make a second copy if that is not an infringement of copyright.

O Be patient. Don't always expect an immediate response. The child may need a little time to process the question.

O Try not to talk at the board whilst writing upon it. It is better to write, turn round, allow a moment for the class to read the information and then explain. Interactive whiteboards, which are becoming a common classroom feature, reduce this problem.

O Avoid making throwaway comments, asides or humorous remarks. These may make the deaf child become confused and demoralised.

O Ask the deaf child questions. They will remain more attentive if you include them in this way. They soon know if you avoid them, and like any child will either use it to their advantage or become disheartened.

O If you ask any child a question, repeat the answer for the benefit of those who haven't heard, using the name of the child you ask. For example:

Billy says that 14 of the elephants were green.
Yes, he's correct.
Rather than
Yes, that's right, and how many were blue?

O Use challenging and stimulating questions and try to stretch the child as you would any other.

O If there is in-class support, acknowledge their presence and role in a positive and open way. (See Chapter 8.)

Managing group discussions

Group discussions, whether large or small, can be a nightmare for a deaf child if strategies and rules are not understood and put into practice by adults and children alike. These are key points to note:

O The child may not be able to locate quickly who is talking.

O What is said may be audible, though not intelligible.

O If more than one person speaks at a time, the deaf child may have problems distinguishing one voice from another.

O If the teacher wears the FM transmitter, it will not pick up voices at a distance.

O The pace can sometimes be too fast for the deaf child to process all the information they receive.

How to help

◉ Devise a way of indicating who is speaking. If you have an FM transmitter, pass it round, allowing each child to speak only when they are holding it. If you don't use a transmitter, you could substitute another object as a classroom management strategy. Don't forget to pass it to the deaf child too.

◉ If the child has speech that is not always easy to understand, establish a positive way of dealing with this. The other children may have fewer problems with understanding than you think. Somehow you have to find this out without embarrassing everyone, and without effectively excluding rather than including. Don't be frightened to ask the child privately.

◉ Ask advice from the ToD or learning support assistant (LSA).

◉ Reflect responses from other pupils (i.e. repeat, if necessary rephrasing).

◉ Identify each speaker's contribution. For example:

Tosepha thinks the giant is wrong, Lee thinks the giant is silly.
What do you think, Billy?
Rather than
Well, that's interesting. What do you think?

Most of this advice is standard good teaching practice, with a few slight variations. Don't expect to adapt your teaching style overnight. The more complex ideas can be built into your approach and management gradually. As you see the benefits of incorporating the strategies, you will be encouraged to try more suggestions. You may notice that the ideas reflect some of the approaches suggested for children with different educational needs. None of the approaches will disadvantage any child, and they may improve overall classroom management and lesson planning.

Getting to know you

A checklist is supplied (Checklist 4) that can be used as the basis of a discussion with a child to get to know more about their hearing difficulty. It may reveal gaps in knowledge, confidence and so on, and identify things that need action. It provides a useful record and should be revisited at least annually as part of the review process.

Checklist 4 – Self-assessment of listening skills

Child: _____ Date: _____

Teacher: _____

1. When did you realise that it was difficult to hear? _____
   _____

2. Does anyone you know have hearing difficulties? _____
   _____

3. Where do you go for a hearing test? _____
   _____

4. Do you have a hearing aid? _____

   Do you wear it: All the time   ☐   Only at home   ☐

   Only at school   ☐   Not very often   ☐

5. Do you like wearing your hearing aid? Why / Why not? _____
   _____

6. Do loud sounds hurt your ears? With/Without hearing aid? _____
   _____

7. Can you tell where a sound is coming from in class? What happens?
   _____

8. Can you hear the door bell or someone knocking? With/Without hearing aid?
   _____

9. Can you use the telephone? Do you have a textphone (minicom) at home?
   _____

10. Whom can you hear best at school? Girls or boys? _____
    _____

11. Do you watch people's faces and lips to help you understand? _____

12. Do you have extra help in school? From whom? Do you like that? _____
    _____

Self-assessment of listening skills

13. Which teachers are easiest to understand? Why?_____
    _____

    If not, why not? When? _____

14. Where do you sit in class? Who decided? Do you think it is the best place to
    hear and see your teacher and classmates?_____
    _____

15. Do you have a special friend who helps you?_____
    _____

16. When you watch a video in school, can you hear what the voices say?_____

    What do you use to help you?_____

17. How do you feel when you do not hear what someone says? _____
    _____

18. Do you tell people when you have not heard them?_____
    _____

19. Do you ever pretend that you have heard when you haven't?_____
    _____

20. Does your hearing difficulty stop you doing anything?_____
    _____

21. How do you behave if someone is nasty to you when you cannot hear?
    _____

22. Is there anything you want changed about your classroom to help you hear
    better or understand lessons better?_____
    _____

23. Is there anything else you are worried about to do with your hearing?
    _____

Action required: _____
_____
_____
_____

Chapter 4
Using residual hearing and amplification

The focus of all environmental and technological management strategies is the enhancement of the reception of a clear and intact acoustic signal.

Carol Flexer (1994),
Facilitating Hearing and Listening in Young Children,
Singular Publishing

Technological management of aids to hearing

This chapter looks at how we can work towards creating a good listening environment. Combined with favourable positioning of key speakers and consistent use of amplification, this will provide the best chance of delivering a clear and intact acoustic signal. We know that sounds must pass through the auditory system to the brain before a child can learn to interpret and understand them. It is vital that we endeavour to enable this process.

Understanding the listening environment

Schools often present demanding and constantly changing listening situations.

Children need an intelligible speech signal if they are to learn the word–sound differences that underlie the development of spoken communication. There are three critical elements in speech intelligibility.

The signal to noise ratio

If the teacher's voice is competing with noise from whatever source, the signal to noise ratio is unfavourable. Background noise can come from talking, heating systems, traffic, televisions, movement of furniture and so on.

- ● People with hearing typically require a signal to noise ration of + 6dB in order to hear intelligible speech.
- ● Children with a hearing loss need a signal to noise ratio of + 20dB.

The average classroom ratio is only +4 or + 5dB, which is less than ideal even for those with normal hearing.

Distance

A child's ability to hear the teacher's voice decreases dramatically towards the back of the room. Audibility decreases as the distance from the speaker increases (about a 6dB drop for every doubling of distance).

The situation is worst for children sitting at the furthest point from the teacher, who may be receiving only 55 per cent of the speech signal. This loss of speech information is highly significant for a hearing impaired child, who won't necessarily have the knowledge and ability to fill in the gap.

Reverberation (echo)

Reverberation affects speech recognition by masking the direct sound energy. Hard walls, high ceilings, glass windows and uncarpeted floors reflect many sounds. As the teacher speaks louder to overcome the echo, the vowels are

One day man will be forced to fight noise as relentlessly as Cholera and the plague.

Robert Koch, discoverer
of the tuberculosis bacillus

emphasised, further obscuring meaning. Reverberation disrupts hearing more than background noise, although background noise is affected by reverberation.

Sound Field System

The Sound Field System (SFS) is a device that improves the speech to noise ratio by the use of a remote microphone placed near the speaker. It ensures that a clearer and more intelligible signal is received by all children, both hearing and deaf. It is a means of amplifying a whole classroom, through the use of two, three or four wall or ceiling mounted loud-speakers. All children, hearing and deaf, benefit from the improved and consistent signal to noise ratio, no matter where the teacher is in the classroom.

The transmitter is worn by the speaker. A signal is transmitted to an amplifier connected to the loud-speakers. The teacher can move about freely as there are no wires connecting them to other parts of the equipment. Pupils do not wear receivers as the sound comes from the loud-speakers and is evenly distributed around the room.

The system is set approximately 10–15dB above the average level of background noise.

Individual portable systems are available and can be taken from class to class.

Other features

The SFS provides a favourable speech to noise ratio for most children, but will not be sufficient for children with severe or profound hearing difficulties. Deaf children who wear an FM radio aid can tune their receiver to the same frequency as the transmitter on the SFS. Problems with SFS are more easily identifiable than those with a hearing aid as everyone in the room can hear whether it is working properly.

Hearing aids

Hearing aids are usually the first piece of technology prescribed for a child with a hearing loss. They enhance the reception of sound through amplification.

Basic facts about hearing aids

- They are like individual public address systems.
- They do not correct the hearing difficulty. They alter the acoustic input by amplifying sounds, then shape them to the individual's auditory potential. Aids can be adjusted to meet the requirements of all types and degrees of hearing loss.
- Hearing aids function best in a quiet environment where the speaker is close to the listener.
- The hearing aid provides access to the auditory environment. It takes a long period of acclimatisation for the child to understand the meaning of incoming sounds.

When acoustic improvements were carried out, the children were able to improve their performance in early reading, learning numbers and their speech ability.

L.E. Maxwell and G.W. Evans (2000), 'The Effects of Noise on Pre-school Children's Reading Skills', *Journal of Environmental Psychology*, 20

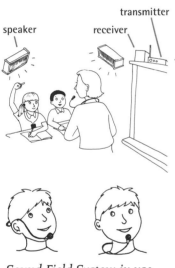

speaker   receiver   transmitter

Sound Field System in use

Hearing aids are described according to where they are worn. In order of decreasing size these categories are: body, spectacle, behind the ear, in the ear, in the canal and completely in the canal.

H. Dillon (2001), *Hearing Aids*, Boomerang Press

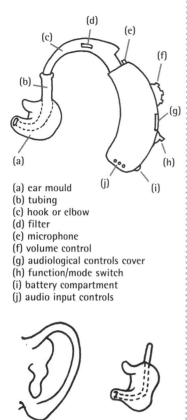

(a) ear mould
(b) tubing
(c) hook or elbow
(d) filter
(e) microphone
(f) volume control
(g) audiological controls cover
(h) function/mode switch
(i) battery compartment
(j) audio input controls

pinna   ear mould

Hearing aid components

Parts of a hearing aid

All hearing aids have the following components:

- Microphone – converts the acoustic signal into an electrical signal.
- Amplifier – shapes the signal, making it louder.
- Battery – provides power for the hearing aid.
- Receiver – converts the amplified and modified signal back into a signal that can be heard.
- Ear mould – directs the sound from the hearing aid directly into the ear. If it does not fit well, it will be inefficient. Feedback or whistling is created when it does not provide an airtight fit. Children need new ear moulds regularly to accommodate the changing sizes and shapes of their growing ears.

Teachers need to feel confident when checking hearing aid function. Young children cannot do this themselves, although the aim is to make them fully independent in all aspects of use, care and maintenance.

Knowing the names of the parts, their functions and how to do basic running repairs will give you confidence and the child will have confidence in you. The most commonly prescribed aids are behind the ear (or post-aurals). They come in a variety of sizes, and children personalise them by choosing their favourite colours for the case and ear moulds.

The microphone is front facing as most of the sound comes from the front. Two aids are generally prescribed for a bilateral loss.

Other types of hearing aid are available, and are prescribed for children in particular circumstances. The National Deaf Children's Society will provide you with additional information, as will any hearing aid manufacturer.

Fault finding

Hearing aids need daily checking. Schools should build in procedures for maintenance –such as battery replacement, alerting the visiting ToD or informing the parents. The hearing aid is a sophisticated piece of equipment and fortunately the most common faults are easily remedied. Anything serious is dealt with by an audiologist or manufacturer.

Start with a simple visual inspection, remembering that if you ask the child with two hearing aids to take them both off, they may not then be able to hear you. Check them one at a time. These are the points to watch:

① Are all switches intact, switched on or on the appropriate settings?
② Is the microphone cover secure and clear?
③ Is the hook (elbow) intact? Is the filter still there?
④ Is the hook secure?

Use a fresh battery for the hearing aid check. Check the battery with a battery tester, if you have one.

⑤ Are the battery contacts clean?

⑥ Is the battery inserted properly?

⑦ Is the battery compartment fully closed?

⑧ Are the audiological controls covered?

⑨ Is the tubing free of twists, cracks and holes?

⑩ Does the tubing fit snugly onto the aid?

⑪ Is the ear mould channel free of wax and moisture?

⑫ Is the tip of the ear mould free of wax?

⑬ Is the ear mould split?

⑭ Is there any discoloration of the ear mould or tubing?

⑮ Are the case screws loose or showing signs of wear?

Listening check

Use a stetoclip, a device for listening to and checking hearing aids. It fits over the tip of the mould or the end of the hook. You will have to remove the ear mould first.

① Set the hearing aid to O.

② Turn the volume control down completely.

③ Put on the stetoclip.

④ Turn the M–T–O (microphone, telecoil, off) switch to M.

⑤ Move the volume control up slowly to check whether the sound gets louder as you increase the volume wheel and softer as you decrease the wheel.

⑥ Are there any sudden jumps in loudness as you turn the wheel?

⑦ Does the wheel turn smoothly?

⑧ Is the sound scratchy as you turn the volume control?

⑨ Check for feedback (whistling).

⑩ Reset the aid correctly before you hand it back.

If you have any doubts, make sure you follow your procedures to get the aid seen by an audiologist or ToD (or other appropriate expert).

Feedback check

Feedback is a whistling, high pitched sound that may occur in the following circumstances:

Cause	Remedy
The ear mould is not correctly inserted into the ear	Show the child how to insert it correctly
Mould no longer fits into the ear	Arrange for a new mould to be made
Tubing detached	Reattach tubing
Split in ear hook	Replace ear hook
Hook is too loose	Replace ear hook
Split in tubing	Replace tubing

Safety issues

○ *Swallowing* – children sometimes swallow hearing aid batteries. If this happens, seek medical help immediately.

○ *Battery explosion* – hearing aid batteries are not rechargeable and should be disposed of with care.

Checklist 5 – Hearing aid check

Name: _____ Date: _____

Completed by: _____

							Hearing aid parts	
Battery and holder	Case screws	Switches	Microphone	Hook (elbow) and tube	Control cover	Ear mould	Remarks	
								Action needed

Useful tools for effecting minor repairs

- Extra batteries – batteries go dead at the most inconvenient times. Keep spares.
- Antiseptic wipes – small, handy cloths for cleaning ear moulds and casings.
- A toothbrush – detach the ear mould from the hearing aid and use the toothbrush with soap and water to clear any wax.
- A battery tester – to check the battery power.
- A tiny screwdriver – for loose screws.
- A wax remover – cleans wax from the ear mould opening. One is often supplied with the hearing aid.
- A puffer bulb – blows water out from inside an ear mould or tubing.

❍ *Noise-induced hearing loss* – continual exposure to high levels of noise through the hearing aid can worsen a hearing loss. The volume should be turned down if the child is going to be in very noisy places.

❍ *Physical impact* – a blow to the head can make the hearing aid case crack, which is very painful. Soft ear moulds are recommended for children.

Assistive listening devices

Despite tremendous technological advances, hearing aids are unable to enhance the signal to noise ratio sufficiently in situations where the speaker is not close to the listener. Children with hearing difficulties who have not yet developed competence in oral language need access to a high-quality auditory signal in order to enhance the signal to noise ratio.

Assistive listening devices are designed to address the problems of noise, distance and reverberation.

The personal FM (radio) system

Most children using hearing aids in school would benefit from the use of a personal FM system. They are often provided for children with severe to profound deafness.

Key facts about the FM system

❍ FM stands for Frequency Modulated Radio Transmission.

❍ It is a personal listening device that comprises a remote microphone worn near the speaker's mouth, a transmitter worn by the speaker, and a receiver worn by the listener.

❍ There are no wires connecting speaker to listener.

❍ The FM transmits and receives on a single frequency.

❍ Each receiver will have a 'common' frequency which can be used with the appropriate transmitter when a speaker needs to talk to a group of radio aid wearers simultaneously. If radio aids are being used in adjacent rooms, they should use different frequencies to prevent cross-over.

❍ It creates a listening situation comparable to a teacher being 20cm from the child at all times.

❍ It can be fitted in conjunction with a hearing aid.

❍ It can be used in conjunction with a cochlear implant.

❍ It can be incorporated into a hearing aid.

❍ Many models are available. An LEA may favour a particular model. Occasionally an LEA will purchase models from different manufacturers to cater for individual children's needs.

❍ The internal/external settings of different models will vary.

❍ FM systems are powered by rechargeable batteries.

❍ The remote microphone can be placed close to (but not on top of) the speaker of a television, video monitor and so on.

○ Mobile phones may sometimes interfere with the functioning of the system, as may other equipment using radio frequencies.

○ Dead spots may occur within the field of the system. Once identified, they should be avoided.

How to use the FM system in school

○ Make sure you understand how it works, where the microphone fits, how to switch it on and so on.

○ Make sure that someone teaches the child the language and vocabulary needed to discuss and report faults and problems. Do not assume the child already knows. At the end of this chapter there are three checklists you can use to record understanding.

○ Ask the ToD for a labelled illustration and a copy of the correct settings to keep in the classroom as an aide-memoire.

○ Use the correct vocabulary to describe the parts; for example, 'Pass me the transmitter please, Dale' is better than 'Where's your box?'

○ Agree a safe place for charging and a routine for the child to collect and return the receiver at the start and end of each day.

○ Organise who is going to do the daily check, how it will be recorded and who will take any action needed.

○ The best place to carry out a listening check is in the environment where the radio aid is to be used. It may pick up interference that is not obvious in the store cupboard where it has been charging.

○ Ask your ToD to demonstrate FM checking and trouble-shooting techniques for your particular model.

○ Ask for a written version of the instructions. Display all procedures in a prominent location, ideally immediately next to or under the charging unit.

○ Agree a procedure for a rapid response if any part of the system is faulty.

○ Agree a procedure for weekends and holidays, including where the equipment will be kept and who will be responsible for having the radio aid charged on the first day of term.

○ Establish what to do if the child is absent. Check how long the batteries stay charged.

In the classroom

○ Teachers talk from the moment they open the classroom door, but the deaf child will not hear you until you have put on and switched on the transmitter. It should be the first thing you do. Even if you are only taking the register before you hurtle off to assembly, switch it on. Some important information is usually given out in the first ten minutes of any session.

○ You may have to think about your clothing. If you wear trousers you can clip the transmitter to your belt. Wearing it round your neck is a favoured option, but if you bend forward you may find that the transmitter crashes into the pencil pots. A little thought about using pockets is helpful.

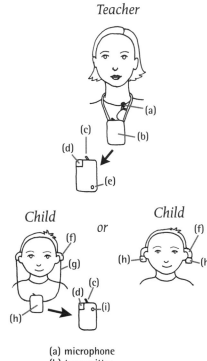

Teacher

Child   *or*   *Child*

(a) microphone
(b) transmitter
(c) on/off
(d) frequency indicator
(e) low battery alert
(f) hearing aids
(g) direct audio input
(h) receiver
(i) light off when receiver switched on

Radio aid in use by child and teacher

○ Clip the microphone to your clothing so that it does not rub against anything or bump into jewellery. All sounds are amplified equally loudly.

○ If you have a visitor who needs to talk to the class, pass the transmitter to them. Don't accept the response 'Oh, it's all right. I'll only be a minute.'

○ Turn the transmitter off if you are speaking privately and at break and so on.

○ Take off the child's system at break or for PE, storing it carefully and safely.

○ If the transmitter has an antenna/aerial, let it hang. Don't fiddle with it.

○ Encourage other children to use the transmitter in a group discussion or when turn taking in reading.

Cochlear implants

A cochlear implant is a device designed to provide sound to children who derive little or no benefit from conventional hearing aids. It is beyond the scope of this book to give more than a brief overview of this complex topic. Surgery is necessary to implant the receiver and electrodes. These parts will not be seen. The external visible parts are the microphone, transmitter and speech processor.

How does it work?

The microphone picks up sound which is sent to the speech processor to be converted to a digital signal. This passes back to the headpiece, through the skin to the receiver, and is delivered to the electrode array to stimulate the auditory nerve. The brain interprets the signal as sound. Cochlear implants can be used in conjunction with a personal FM system.

There will be a team of support staff for a child who has an implant and their family. The local ToD will be an important part of the team and will probably be the individual with whom you establish the most regular contact. This is particularly true as the child gets older and the involvement from the Cochlear Implant Centre where the device was fitted reduces.

Most centres produce their own materials specifically designed for teachers working with the child needing support to develop their listening skills. Guidelines for working with children with cochlear implants are available from the BATOD website (see *Useful contacts* on page 64).

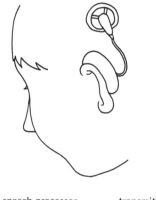

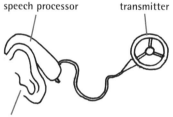

speech processor   transmitter

pinna

Cochlear implant component parts

Checklist 6 – Parts of behind-the-ear hearing aid

Parts of hearing aid	Can point to it when asked	Can understand when used in context by adult	Can say the word in context with prompting	Can say in context without prompting
	Date	Date	Date	Date
Ear mould				
Tube				
Elbow (hook)				
Battery				
Case				
Switch				
Volume control				
Battery compartment				
Microphone				
Controls				

You can use this format to record competence in other related areas, e.g. reporting faulty equipment.

Checklist 7 – Parts of radio aid receiver

Parts of radio aid receiver	Can point to it when asked	Can understand when used in context by adult	Can say the word in context with prompting	Can say in context without prompting
	Date	Date	Date	Date
Battery				
On/Off switch				
Green light (transmission indicator)				
Red light (reception and battery indicator)				
Built-in microphone				
Cover				
Frequency control				
Charging contact				
Remote microphone				
Clip				
Bi-lead				
Shoe				
Output hole for the connection of bi-lead				
Charger				
Plug				
Wire				

Checklist 8 – Parts of radio aid transmitter

Parts of the radio aid transmitter	Can point to it when asked	Can understand when used in context by adult	Can say the word in context with prompting	Can say in context without prompting
	Date	Date	Date	Date
Battery				
On/Off switch				
Red light (battery indicator)				
Built-in microphone				
Cover				
Frequency control				
Microphone				
Clip				
Harness				
Satellite microphone				
Microphone clip				

Chapter 5
Strategies for developing literacy and numeracy

Literacy

Children who can hear without difficulty approach the challenges of literacy armed with sustained experience of a vast and complex language system. They arrive at the task of writing when they have something to write about, something they have already spoken about and heard many times. With so much spoken language at their disposal, when they learn to read they are already familiar with the words in the text. The task is to decode the spidery squiggles.

If a child cannot hear properly, they may not have the levels of spoken language skill necessary to approach literacy with confidence. It is important that their level of conceptual understanding is known. Children often comprehend situations, but are unable to communicate well about them. Alternatively, children who appear to have excellent communication skills may have poor spoken conversational ability. Children may be very adept at disguising gaps in their knowledge and understanding.

Specific difficulties

The most startling difficulty may be the vast gaps in knowledge and awareness of language. You may find that a child is not familiar with a common piece of vocabulary or particular term. Remember that we only know words we have learnt through use. If a child has not had experience of good-quality, consistent input, they may not know some quite basic language. It is a mistake to assume they cannot learn. They still have intact potential and experience, and explanation will do a lot to make up for delay.

Becoming 'deaf aware' will help you identify situations which are unhelpful for a child with hearing difficulties. For instance, seeing other people talking and communicating only shows how it is done. A child with normal hearing will be able to listen, hear and watch, gaining reinforcing exposure to spoken language. It is not easy to predict what a deaf child will make of such a situation. Without an explanation, connected events such as a parent leaving the room and returning with letters may appear magical to a child who hasn't heard the letters dropping on the mat. There are many situations which may lead to similar confusion. Deaf children often seem naïve because of this lack of understanding.

A child's writing will reflect the structure of their spoken language and will often reveal the level of competence, ability and misunderstanding. For example:

- ◗ omitting word endings;
- ◗ omitting s from plurals;

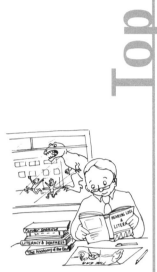

"Reading around the subject can be very absorbing."

Top tips

For literacy

- Read around the subject of deafness and literacy. It is impossible to do much more here than raise awareness. Sources of much valuable information and advice can be found in the *Resources* and *Useful contacts* sections (see pages 63–64).
- Establish the level of conceptual understanding of each individual child so that they can be appropriately stimulated by the choice of suitable reading material.
- Establish the developmental language level of each child so that you know the complexity of sentences understood and used.
- If a child cannot hear properly they will have difficulty recognising phonemes and morphemes. If they can be encouraged to recognise whole words visually and derive meaning from context, they are likely to be more successful.
- When correcting work, make sure you know which are hearing errors (e.g. omitting high-frequency sounds such as *s* and *sh*). That may mean you need to explain that they are present even though they cannot be heard.
- Use familiar words for phonic work rather than teaching new vocabulary through phonics.
- Try to work with syllables rather than isolated phonemes.
- Remember that the deaf child may need to look at you, the book and/or the board. Learn how to accommodate this reference triangle.
- If a child does not have enough hearing to follow video tapes successfully, provide a book which follows the script. This will help them develop an understanding of reading and gain vicarious experience.
- If using a Big Book, provide a small copy for use by the teaching assistant (TA) or community support worker (CSW).
- Remember to consider the quality of the listening environment.
- Ensure the amplification technology is working at all times.
- Use the home–school book to provide information about experiences that will provide and reinforce new vocabulary.
- Ensure that the child and the TA/CSW are in a comfortable and appropriate position that is well established and recognised by all. It is worth explaining that a child reliant on lip reading cannot do so from the back of the group.
- Do not use linguistic short cuts, which may help avoid a potential misunderstanding but may consolidate bad habits in the child.
- Be sure you can identify unusual structures in a child's spoken or written language, and be aware that normal developmental structures may be delayed.
- Know and understand normal development structures for children using BSL.
- If you correct work, discuss the corrections with the child and ask them to read the corrected version back to you. You could then read the corrected version back to them or ask them to write out the corrected work again to reinforce the learning.

- ❍ mixing tenses;
- ❍ confusing word order;
- ❍ confusion of homonyms (e.g. *their/there*);
- ❍ omitting function words that are not stressed in running speech;
- ❍ confusion or lack of knowledge of parts of the verb *to be – am, was, have been*;

◆ absence of auxiliary verbs – *would/will*;

◆ little knowledge of prosodic features of spoken language;

◆ little knowledge of features that belong only in the written form.

Numeracy

Factors that might cause children with a permanent hearing loss to experience difficulties acquiring numeracy skills include the following:

◆ Limited access to incidental mathematical talk, particularly during the pre-school years.

◆ Lack of auditory experience may have an impact on short-term memory skills and increase response time for addition and subtraction tasks.

◆ Mathematical language is particularly challenging because of the complexity of mathematical semantics and syntax.

◆ Mathematical problems are often presented with little or no context.

◆ The early introduction of mental arithmetic in the numeracy strategy presents problems to children who cannot hear properly even when using amplification.

◆ The pace and rigour of whole-class numeracy sessions may cause deaf children to struggle as they need additional time to 'tune in' to the content of a lesson and to process information before they can respond.

◆ The phonological similarity of some mathematical vocabulary can be confusing (e.g. 18 and 80 sound similar and have identical lip patterns).

Top tips

For numeracy

• Involve the ToD, TA and/or CSW in all aspects of the planning process.

• Make use of the strong visual element of mathematics whenever you can to illuminate meaning (e.g. make frequent use of a number line, 100 square, pictures, diagrams, graphs, computer programmes and games – for which the rules are picked up quickly by watching a demonstration).

• During any whole-class oral work, ask support staff to position themselves close to any children who need special help.

Oral work and mental calculation

◆ *Seating position.* The hearing-impaired child should have a good view of the teacher's face and the faces of other children in order to follow the lip patterns of the speaker. It is important that the teacher does not have their back to a window, as in bright sunlight their facial features may be invisible.

◆ *Accessing contributions from other children.* The teacher can help the child with hearing difficulties access speech by repeating other children's contributions. The spoken word can be reinforced by the written word.

◆ *Teaching in parallel.* There may be times when the hearing-impaired pupil will need to be taught in parallel to the class. The child will need to be withdrawn to a quiet environment. The number of times that this is needed will depend upon the level of the pupil's language development.

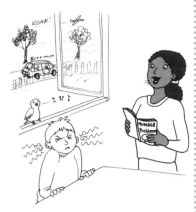

Main teaching activity

This covers whole-class, group, paired and individual work.

- *Reinforce instructions.* Instructions need to be reinforced, and a check made to make sure that the child understands the requirements of the task.
- *Using the radio aid.* If a child uses a radio aid, the microphone should be passed around or the radio transmitter used as a conference microphone during group or paired work.
- *Background noise.* The hearing-impaired child will have difficulty accessing information if the level of ambient noise is high.

The plenary session

- *Include the hearing-impaired child.* Include contributions from the hearing-impaired child, even if the work has been undertaken during parallel sessions and/or the child's speech is not clear.
- *Using the radio aid.* When the children are reporting back to the class, use the radio microphone so that the hearing-impaired child has a greater chance of accessing the children's speech.
- *Repeat key points.* The hearing-impaired child will have a better chance of retaining knowledge if key points are repeated during the plenary session.

Teach the semantics of mathematics

Pay attention to the following:

- everyday words that have a more exact meaning when used mathematically (e.g. similar, difference, divide, table, altogether, rounded);
- specialised terms (multiplication, factor, denominator);
- combined concepts (least common multiple);
- English terms with verb particles (divided by / divided into);
- inference (e.g. the term 'the number' / 'a number' in 'five times the number 6 is three more than 9 times a number');
- different terms referring to a single mathematical operation (less, take away, subtract, minus).

Teach English syntactic structures used in mathematics:

- for example, word order (e.g. $8 \div 2$ can be thought of as 'How many lots of 2 are there in 8?');
- logical connectors (e.g. if ... then, either ... or);
- comparatives (e.g. as tall as, Usha is older than Jack, greater/less than).

Chapter 6
Communication options

A variety of communication options are available to deaf children. Like children with normal hearing, they are entitled to develop a communication system which enables them to function comparably and effectively in all settings and for all purposes. For the majority of children with hearing difficulties in school, the approach used will be based on English. Many will choose to use a sign system in conjunction with amplification. Some may use BSL as their main route to communication while developing literacy skills through written English.

The decision to adopt one method in preference to another is arrived at after lengthy discussion between all professionals and family members involved in the support of the child.

Auditory–oral approaches

This term describes all the approaches used to promote the acquisition of spoken language. The effective use of residual hearing and other appropriate amplification is essential, and signing is not used. It includes an emphasis on lip reading and the production of intelligible speech by the child, and is a visual approach to the acquisition of spoken and written English.

Natural auralism

Natural auralism is an auditory–oral approach that takes children along a similar path to thc acquisition of language to the one a hearing child treads, learning through interaction and meaningful conversation.

Approaches incorporating a signed component
Total Communication

The Total Communication (TC) approach, through the medium of English, involves using a combination of signed and auditory/oral components. The sign components include:

- ● fingerspelling;
- ● sign-supported English;
- ● signed English;
- ● Makaton vocabulary;
- ● cued speech.

Each component may be used alone or in combination with another. You should be provided with advice about how best to use support to meet the child's needs.

Total Communication
The child will be supported by adults who will help to provide:
 sign supported English;
 and/or
 signed English;
 and/or
 cued speech;
 and/or
 BSL.

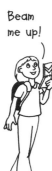

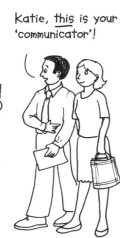

Sign bilingualism

This approach uses British Sign Language (BSL), the language of the deaf community. It has its own grammatical structure and linguistic features, and cannot be used simultaneously with spoken English. Children educated using BSL learn English as an additional language. In a mainstream setting, a communicator/interpreter will be necessary.

Opportunities to learn the appropriate signed approach to help you communicate effectively with the child should be sought. It may be possible for the children in your class/school to learn some sign from an appropriate person. If a child is using sign bilingualism, you will be supported by a ToD and/or a CSW, who are qualified to provide a silent, simultaneous interpretation of whatever is being taught and to relay a voiced interpretation of the deaf child's contributions.

In-class support

Most teachers are very experienced at working with other adults in the classroom to support children with special needs. The level of support provided for deaf children varies, depending on the nature and degree of difficulty that an individual may be experiencing or be expected to experience in a mainstream setting.

The adults who work in this role may be there to:
- check that the child's hearing aids are working;
- ensure that the personal FM system is working;
- check that the child has understood instructions and messages;
- keep a record of work covered;
- modify the language used by the teacher if this has not been understood;
- note areas of confusion or uncertainty;
- plan sessions to target areas of confusion;
- provide notes and written records for the child to use;
- monitor how well a child is performing in class;
- signal who is speaking in a question-and-answer session;
- provide an explanation of what is happening out of earshot (a hearing child might be able to overhear information which is to their advantage educationally);
- provide information for the class teacher and visiting ToD to help in targeted future teaching opportunities, reviews, assessments and so on;
- provide encouragement to develop independent learning skills;
- provide encouragement to develop relationships independently;
- provide opportunities for privacy, and even for naughtiness and laziness.

If a sign interpreter fills the in-class support role, their function will be different. The sign interpreter will be there to translate from English to BSL or Sign

Support for English. It is not an interpreter's role to explain or re-teach the lesson content. They facilitate access and communication.

If you are expecting a ToD, CSW or LSA to support a child in your class, you may be feeling apprehensive. It is well worth the effort of making some basic preparation. Checklist 9 will help.

If you have read the previous chapters, you will know which questions you need to ask.

Adults often react badly when confronted by someone whose speech they do not understand. Some find it so embarrassing that they avoid talking directly to that person again. This is a normal, but unfortunate, reaction.

If you want to foster a positive attitude to the deaf child in your class, you must demonstrate one yourself. If you take evasive action, so will the class.

To find suddenly after years of talking, teaching and instructing that not only will you not be understood, but that the child looks away for an interpretation from someone else, may affect your self-esteem and create feelings of resentment or irritation. Again, this is a normal reaction. Remember that it will show in your face, and the child with a hearing difficulty looks closely at faces for information.

Before you encounter this situation in class, read the guidance provided in Chapter 3, which will help you prepare for the effective inclusion of children with all levels of hearing difficulty. Try to arrange to watch another teacher in another school where deaf children are included. You will then see what you have read being put into practice.

Checklist 9 – Questions before meeting the deaf child

1. What type and degree of hearing loss do they have?
2. When was it diagnosed? How old were they then?
3. Is it bilateral?
4. Is it the same in both ears?
5. Do they wear hearing aids all the time at school?
6. Do they have a cochlear implant? If so, when was this done?
7. Does the child use a personal FM radio system? If so, who will provide training in its use?
8. Do they have intelligible speech?
9. Do they have good lip-reading skills?
10. Which signing system do they use in school, if any?
11. Do they sign at home? Are the parents deaf or hearing?
12. Does the child have other deaf family members?
13. Is English the first language in their home?
14. How would you describe their nature and personality?
15. How much in-class support will be provided? Will it be one person or shared?
16. How much time will the ToD be spending with the child? When? What for?
17. Whom do I contact when I need help?
18. What additional training will be available?
19. Will written guidance and additional sources of information be offered?
20. Who else works with the child on a regular basis?
21. Does the child have any other special needs?
22. Does the child have any health problems that might affect their learning?
23. Could I meet or observe the child in another setting before they join the class?
24. What do I tell the class?
25. How do I introduce the interpreter?
26. What is deaf awareness?

Chapter 7
Deaf awareness across the curriculum

Deaf awareness

Any school endeavouring to include deaf children successfully should have a thorough understanding of the term 'deaf awareness'. Deaf awareness should be a distinct part of any special needs policy, subject to the regular reviews, checking, revising and analysis undergone for any school policy that informs the daily practice of both adults and children.

Deaf awareness is not a once-and-only training experience. It builds on skills, knowledge and experience. It needs to be continually reviewed and explored. This is a challenging prospect for any school, particularly as deafness is a low-incidence condition in school. However, it is worth the effort and makes a huge difference to the success of any programme of inclusion.

Deafness is a low-incidence disability. That does not mean that it is of low importance. You will need to fight your corner to ensure that higher-incidence special needs do not dominate the training packages.

Who is it for?

Deaf awareness is relevant to all adults and all children within the school environment who come into contact with deaf children in school, for however brief a time. Lunchtime supervisors, school secretaries, site supervisors, taxi drivers and escorts are all significant members of the school, as are parents and siblings of the children. The importance of their impact on a deaf child's social and emotional development cannot be overestimated.

Who delivers it?

There are certificated training courses available through the Council for the Advancement of Communication with Deaf People (CACDP). There are formal modules within sign language courses. There are also informal courses run by members of the deaf community, as well as Inset packages run by special needs services using deaf tutors and role models. This is not something that an inexperienced school can be expected to do without help and guidance. The National Deaf Children's Society (NDCS) produces a range of relevant publications and schools can now sign up to the NDCS's ten-point Deaf Friendly Schools Pledge, which aims to help schools become more accessible for deaf children.

What does it contain?

A good deaf awareness course will contain information and guidance on:

- understanding the barriers that limit opportunities;
- positive action and behaviours that will reduce and reverse discrimination;
- understanding how deafness affects communication;

- understanding and identifying the different forms of communication;
- a knowledge of basic tactics that assist communication;
- the development and demonstration of a positive attitude;
- understanding the cultural differences between groups who use BSL and/or spoken language;
- a knowledge of the technical aids available;
- resources and useful contacts.

How will this help the deaf child?

Feelings of isolation are all too common in children with hearing difficulties. Gaps in social skills and emotional immaturity can easily result from being misunderstood, overlooked and 'separate'. The more information available for those working and living alongside the deaf child, the more informed their behaviour and attitude will be. This will lead to a more contented, happier child who is more likely to learn.

Social and emotional needs

Deaf children have the same social and emotional needs as other children. They have specific additional needs because of the impact a hearing loss has on their experience of the world.

Factors affecting social and emotional development

Early development of emotional literacy is important for every child. A large part of their understanding of their own and other people's emotions is learnt through conversation. In addition, children acquire an understanding of what other people are thinking and feeling by talking about what they believe other people might be thinking. Deaf children may lack experience in these areas if, when they start to demonstrate difficulties with speech and language, emphasis is placed on areas of language development such as those vital to communicate on a daily basis. As the child grows older, they may also lack the opportunities for the incidental learning that is essential for continuing emotional maturity.

Children need to have an understanding of their own identity as a deaf individual, and to be comfortable with it. They need to accept and to understand their deafness. How they are treated by others because of their deafness is a defining element of a deaf identity.

Contact with other deaf children and adults may be very limited if a deaf child is in a mainstream setting. A deaf child needs to experience deaf role models as well as role models with normal hearing.

Checklist 10 – Are you deaf aware?

Try answering these questions.

1. How many people in the UK are affected by hearing loss?

2. Why is 'hearing impaired' an unacceptable term to some people?

3. How many deaf people in the UK use sign language?

4. What is positive body language? Can you demonstrate it?

5. List the barriers to access in your school for children with hearing difficulty.

6. How could you gain a deaf child's attention when they are out of earshot?

7. What are the benefits of the Disability Discrimination Act (DDA) for deaf children?

8. How does your school ensure that the acoustic environment is suitable for a child with a cochlear implant?

9. What help can a deaf parent expect from your school?

10. How many adults in your school have a hearing difficulty?

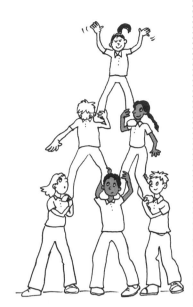

"Design activities in which pupils work together co-operatively."

That Billy is always trying to grab my hearing aids.

Sam, aged 7

I get fed up of being called 'deafie! deafie!'

Gurpreet, aged 8

What can be done?

① Create situations involving social interactions to help the pupils' self-esteem and to help them develop a positive state of mind.

② Design activities in which pupils work together co-operatively, then discuss with them the nature of the co-operative skills they used.

③ Model effective social behaviour and encourage pupils to talk about particular situations and discuss how people might feel in those situations.

④ Explore structured opportunities for deaf children to meet other deaf children socially. Even a child wearing one hearing aid for a moderate unilateral loss will benefit from knowing that they are not the only child with hearing problems.

⑤ Explore opportunities for deaf children to meet, both socially and formally, successful deaf adults who can be role models. It is important that they experience older people functioning in employment and learning environments, and have the opportunity to develop appropriate relationships with them.

⑥ Adapt your PSHE programme to reflect issues likely to be of particular relevance for a child with hearing difficulties.

Bullying

All schools endeavour to implement an anti-bullying policy. Where there are children with hearing difficulties, their particular circumstances need to be acknowledged in the guidance. Not all deaf children are bullied, but they are frequently vulnerable to bullying in the school environment and they are often at a disadvantage because of poor listening conditions, possibly combined with speech and communication difficulties. The indicators of bullying are familiar to most school staff. Deaf children will manifest the same behaviours as others. However, they may be overlooked because they do not have the opportunity to voice their concerns. It is also possible that such a child will not have the language needed to discuss their concerns or fears. They may need considerably more time to explain what is happening and to understand what is relevant and why. For instance, a deaf child may not be able to take part in a small group discussion in which an adult is trying to get the story straight. Indeed, putting a vulnerable child into such a situation may result in the unintentional support of bullying behaviour.

Prevention

Willingness to take bullying seriously is at the heart of every successful prevention strategy:

❍ Make time available for children to discuss their concerns.

❍ Regularly review the policy, checking that the needs of vulnerable groups are acknowledged and understood.

❍ Ensure that deaf children understand the procedures and opportunities open to them.

❍ Ensure that active communication is maintained with home. This is particularly important for a child with poor communication skills, who may rely on the significant intervention of adults.

◗ Demonstrate a positive attitude towards deafness in the classroom. Children need to experience respect for diversity, not the disrespect of difference.

◗ Include deaf-awareness training for all as part of an ongoing, inclusive approach to anti-bullying and anti-harassment.

Child protection

It will take longer than usual to get to know a child with poor speech or one who uses BSL. Consequently, less-experienced adults may miss clues or incidental disclosures that are easy to spot amongst children with normal hearing who are engaged in classroom activities. The CSW or TA may be the adult most likely to express their concerns first.

The child protection policy and procedures must be known to and understood by all involved with children in school. Without joined-up thinking, a shared and consistent approach to recording, monitoring and reporting, there is significant potential for serious misunderstanding and harm.

Independent learning

We have looked at methods you can use to ensure that a child with a hearing loss is not further disadvantaged. One of the most important things you can do is to encourage the child to take responsibility for their own learning and hearing difficulties.

Children with hearing loss do not automatically understand the impact of their hearing problems. They need to be talked to about why you are sitting them in a particular spot, why you are always trying to face them, and why you attract their attention before speaking.

They will not automatically know the names of the parts of their hearing aid. Nor will they be able to report faults adequately unless they are taught how. The expectation is that the child will be able to participate to some degree in the use and maintenance of their hearing aid. Maximum independence is the goal; consequently strategies have to be devised and targets set. Your visiting ToD will be able to give you help and advice with this.

It takes time for a child to work things out. The breakthrough will come when they, for instance, approach you independently and ask to change their seating position because their better ear is facing the open window and the gardener is mowing the lawn. You will recognise a significant moment when the deaf child asks you to repeat something because you were facing the board when you spoke. Your first reaction might be to feel criticised, but if you take a moment to reflect you will see that it is much easier to meet children's needs when they tell you exactly what they are.

Once I'm in that swimming pool, I can't hear a thing.

Wayne, aged 8

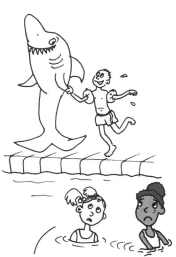

I'm not sure about Valon's new buddy!

The other boys get mad if I don't hear them tell me to pass the football.

Kevin, aged 12

Specific subjects

Swimming

Once a child who normally wears hearing aids takes them off, they cannot hear as well as other children. They must remove them for swimming and leave them somewhere safe and dry. Once in the water, they will not be able to hear shouted instructions.

If the child is swimming away from you, they may not respond to your whistle or your shouts. It is usual to appoint a buddy who alerts the deaf child when they need to stop and pay attention. The buddy will be close to the deaf child in the water and will explain what the teacher/instructor is saying. It is good practice not to use the same buddy always. As an exercise in deaf awareness this is very valuable. The buddy quickly learns how to cope with unfavourable listening conditions and establish good communication. Relationships that might not normally present themselves in the classroom are often forged in these situations.

Sport

Generally, hearing aids are removed for sporting activities as:

- they are not efficient over distance;
- they fall off easily if a wearer is running or involved in vigorous exercise;
- they can easily be damaged or lost;
- any collision may force the aid and mould against the head, which is very painful.

It may be necessary to prepare children for new games or the introduction of rules. For example, a deaf child standing on a field trying to listen to an explanation of the rules of football when not wearing hearing aids is unlikely to understand much. If they are also unable to hear team members shouting instructions as they play, they will be even less likely to be considered a valuable member of the team.

The message therefore is to be aware and inventive. If it is possible to anticipate a problem, then all should be done to alleviate any likely disadvantage for the child. Children with cochlear implants are generally advised to avoid contact sports.

Music

There is no reason why children with hearing difficulties should not take an active role in the production and appreciation of music – in fact, many respond very well to this area of the curriculum. Although deaf children may need more structured opportunities to discover the instruments that best suit their hearing abilities, personality and temperament, they, like all children, can gain musical experience through many routes. Considerable practical advice is available from specialists in music for the deaf. A useful contact is listed on page 64.

Chapter 8
Supporting roles

Professional support

Here is a list of some of the individuals and agencies involved with deaf children and their families throughout their lives. There are others with whom you will be familiar; those are not included here.

- ENT consultant surgeon – usually hospital based. Responds to referrals from Senior Clinical Medical Officer (SCMO) and audiologists. May prescribe medication and perform corrective surgery.

- Audiologist – person with in-depth knowledge of hearing, acoustics and balance. Has rehabilitative and diagnostic role.

- Audiological scientist – usually hospital based. Responsible for identification and rehabilitation of hearing and balance disorders.

- Educational audiologist – usually a teacher of the deaf with an additional qualification in educational audiology or audiological science. Usually works within LEA support services to provide support for children and families, ensuring optimum amplification and use of residual hearing. They provide written advice for the Code of Practice assessment.

- Teacher of the Deaf (ToD) / consultant teacher – specialises in working with deaf children. Works in a variety of situations including schools, homes and clinics.

- Social worker for the deaf – social worker with special training not only in generic social work, but also in the special needs of deaf people. They have the skills necessary to communicate using a variety of methods in a variety of situations.

- Advocate – usually a member of an independent team that provides individual support to deaf people and their families.

- Educational psychologist – part of an LEA team with special understanding of how children think and behave. They typically visit schools to see children with difficulties and advise staff and parents on a course of action. They are involved in the preparation of advice for special needs Code of Practice stages.

- Speech and language therapist – works with children who have difficulty in producing speech sounds. They help deaf children use residual hearing and speech. Some are employed by the NHS, some in independent practice and some in schools funded by the LEA.

- Communication support worker (CSW) – person trained to support deaf children in schools/colleges. Trained in communication skills, deaf issues and teaching methods.

- LEA officer – provides parents with information, help and advice relating to their particular situation within the education system as it relates to the special needs Code of Practice, rights and responsibilities.

Effective liaison presupposes a clear understanding of the role of the diverse professional agencies involved in the support of a deaf pupil in a mainstream school.

RNID (2000), *Effective Inclusion of Deaf Pupils in Mainstream Schools*

◗ Deaf role model / tutor – a deaf person who will work with children and families to provide advice, information, communication training and counselling.

◗ Cochlear implant team – group of audiologists, teachers, scientists, medical and administrative personnel that supports family and child throughout the stages of assessment, surgery and habilitation for a cochlear implant.

The LEA's special needs advisory services will have a team of ToDs who are generally recognised as the co-ordinators of the relevant information in respect of school and education issues.

Levels of involvement

The more severe the impact of the hearing difficulty, the more contact you are likely to have from other agencies. If the child has a Statement of SEN, the levels and type of involvement will be clearly explained on the statement and contact will be easily established.

In an LEA where the funding for the special needs advisory teams has been delegated to schools, you may have to pay for ToD involvement for children not in possession of a statement. It is unlikely that you will have contact from a ToD to monitor children with Glue Ear. Your school may decide to buy in a training package from the advisory service on an annual basis as this is a common problem in Years 1–5.

A child does not automatically receive regular support because they are wearing a hearing aid. The LEA will have provided clear guidelines for each school on levels and types of involvement available. You will probably find you will have to be creative about how you achieve effective and efficient contact with the advisory service. A regular audit of the training needs and special needs in your school will show up the areas of development.

Speech and language therapy

Deaf children do not automatically receive speech and language therapy. It depends on individual need. If the child has additional special needs, this will affect the type and level of involvement. Most speech and language therapists are employed by the NHS. A few work independently, for LEAs, in special schools or for charitable organisations.

If the child has a statement and speech therapy involvement is mentioned, be aware that if it is listed in Part 3 the LEA is responsible for funding. If it is in Parts 5 and 6, it is non-educational provision.

Speech and language therapy may be provided in or out of school. It may be delivered by a speech therapist or by a ToD or TA following a programme written by a speech therapist.

If you have a concern about a child who is finding it especially hard to develop language and communication skills, you should be able to refer directly to a speech and language therapist through the school SENCo.

Working with communication support workers and interpreters

In the support and education of a child with hearing difficulties, you will be expected to work and liaise with specialists. Some you will meet periodically, and some will be involved in your classroom on a day-to-day basis. It may initially be challenging to assimilate these new personnel into your teaching style and routine, but they will soon come to enrich your classroom experience and skills. Together you can create a rewarding teaching environment for the child with hearing difficulties, and indeed the whole class.

What to expect

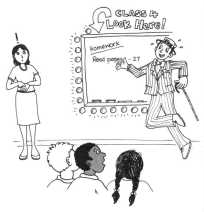

"You may have to draw the class's attention to board work, but they will adapt quickly."

● Initially the children without hearing difficulties will be fascinated and distracted by signing. It soon passes, and it doesn't stop them listening to you. The most disconcerting aspect may be that all eyes will be facing away from you. Just carry on teaching. You may have to draw the class's attention to board work, but they will adapt quickly. Once all eyes are back on you, it is easy to overlook the one child looking at the interpreter. As you become deaf aware, you will be able to indicate by voice or gesture when you want the deaf child to look at you or what you are doing. The interpreter responds to your voice, the deaf child to your gesture. As the deaf child grows older and more experienced, they will use peripheral vision more effectively. You could develop a particular way of standing to indicate that you want visual attention.

● The interpreter will become used to your teaching delivery style and will also anticipate and be alert to your intentions. They will need to be in a position that enables the deaf child to look easily from one of you to the other. This can be inhibiting to start with, but with an open relationship and prior discussion it will improve. If you are a room pacer, you will quickly become aware that the interpreter may find it necessary to follow you.

● All contributions will be interpreted, be they from other children, people popping their head around the door or your asides to yourself. Anything that can be heard by a hearing child will be signed so as not to disadvantage the deaf child.

● When you speak, there will usually be a time lag of anything from a few seconds to half a minute. This doesn't mean that you should slow down your normal rate – that interferes with normal rhythm and meaning. Speak as normal. If you stop speaking and wait for the interpreter to stop signing, the deaf child will probably look at you, expecting a teaching point – as will the interpreter, who may be surprised that you have stopped.

● If you ask a deaf child a question, remember that the child will look to the interpreter for the question, and then at you to answer. You ask the question of the child, not the interpreter – for example, 'Imran, what is the capital of Peru?', not 'Oh, Marie, ask Imran what the capital of Peru is.'

● Allow the child a moment after the interpretation of your question to assimilate or process the information before expecting an answer.

● If a joke is told by you or a pupil, there will be a delay in its being relayed, and the deaf child's response will come later than that of their classmates.

● When the deaf child answers your question, the interpreter will 'voice over' — that is, speak aloud, with the answer in the first person.

● If the deaf child wants to ask a question, they ask you, not the interpreter.

● The interpreter has only one voice or pair of hands, and cannot interpret for more than one person at a time. Group discussions need to be orderly, with one person speaking at a time.

● Interpreting is very demanding physically and mentally. They will need breaks in delivery, which you should plan for.

● Interpreters need advance warning of what you plan to teach. Effective collaboration results from sharing information and good communication. Letting the interpreter know topic, concepts and key vocabulary to be covered each term is a huge help. Interpreters may need time to research individual signs with which they are not familiar.

● Leaving the interpreter literally in the dark when using a video or slides will be disastrous. Remember also that you will need to allow a fraction longer for the deaf child to look at the slide, then the interpreter — sometimes even the interpreter needs an extra moment to look too.

● Further information can be obtained from your ToD or through CACDP.

Effective and efficient liaison

Communicating information amongst all adults working in school is one of the great challenges of education. Employ whichever method works in your school.

Liaison is ongoing and needs to be built into school policy and practice, not added on as an afterthought. Usually add-ons are the first to go under pressure. There is no doubt that without the agreed designated time slot, which should be agreed and valued, effective liaison will not happen.

A simple written agreement is a useful starting point for effective collaboration. It can provide a basis for initial discussion and an easily accessible record of shared and individual roles/responsibilities.

Colleagues who may accept a child leaving a lesson for a violin lesson may not be quite as understanding if a deaf child claims to be going to the medical room to have their radio FM system balanced.

Top tips

Share your skills, knowledge, expertise, planning and records
- Provide colleagues with copies of schemes of work and any planning as part of your weekly routine.
- Provide copies of worksheets, textbooks and so on as part of your daily routine.
- Allow staff to borrow key textbooks. Ideally, provide them with planning information and textbooks well in advance.

Acknowledge and respect the skills of others
- Admit your uncertainty or lack of knowledge and ask for advice.
- Make written observations and notes or queries relating to situations that have arisen in class, so they can be discussed in planned liaison sessions.
- Make opportunities to shadow other professionals.

Building relationships
- Invest effort into building a relationship with the deaf child or children.
- Don't take the relationships you have with other professionals for granted.

Establish shared procedures
- Agree a location where you can leave and exchange information for regular visitors / support staff (e.g. a pigeon hole in the staff room).
- Have simple, clear procedures on dealing with homework, bullying, behaviour and so on that are agreed, written down and adhered to by all concerned.

Keep up to date with developments
- Use the resources available on the Internet to keep you up to date.
- Take up opportunities to accompany professionals on training and Inset.
- Invite professionals to join your training opportunities.

Conclusion

The more you read about deafness and the more experience you have of children with hearing difficulties, the more determined you will become to explore the subject to even greater depth. Both you and the children you teach are bound to benefit from the increased knowledge and confidence you have gained from reading this book.

There are many sources of help and much information to be gained from the vast number of people and agencies committed to the education of deaf children. There have always been contentious issues within this field and no one group has the answers to all the questions. However, there has been exciting progress in many areas over the last 30 years. You will find this an excellent time to start the journey.

Checklist 11 – Agreement

Name of pupil: _____

SN advisory team member(s): _____

School: _____

Contact in school: _____

Number of ToD sessions per week: _____

Start date: _____ Finish date: _____

National Curriculum area – Pre KS 1 2 3 4

Roles and responsibilities

The Support Service for _____ will endeavour to do the following:

1. Check the working of the personal hearing aids and offer advice and information on liaison with Department of Audiology.
2. Check the working of the radio aid and replace or repair as necessary.
3. Provide an explanation verbally and in writing of how the radio aid works, can be checked and is best used.
4. Inform relevant staff of the range of educational implications for any hearing loss of any individual pupil.
5. Respond to Inset requests and keep the school informed about Inset available.
6. Devise work in response to immediate/changing needs.
7. Respond to requests made by the school for consolidation/reinforcement work with pupil.
8. Keep the school informed of any change relating to the child's hearing loss.
9. Facilitate home–school links in connection with matters relating to hearing loss.
10. Take part in all stages of the annual review process as required.
11. Attend case conferences/meetings as required.
12. Make planning documents available as required.
13. Provide termly assessment summaries.
14. Make any results of standardised testing and so on available.
15. Inform the school when a visit has to be cancelled/postponed.

Agreement

The school will endeavour to do the following:

1. Inform the service when the pupil is absent if a visit to the child is planned.
2. Inform the Department of Audiology, educational audiologist and parents when the child's personal hearing aids are not working.
3. Alert the service when the child's radio aid is not working (if applicable).
4. Provide a secure area for charging the radio aid (if applicable).
5. Provide a quiet area where possible/necessary.
6. Alert the service to any changes in a pupil's timetable affecting service support.
7. Invite the teacher of the deaf to take part in all aspects of the annual review process.
8. Provide the service with copies of all relevant documentation.
9. Make available schemes of work / planning sheets and so on.
10. Make opportunities for staff to liaise and plan with the support teacher.
11. Support the service's attempts to co-ordinate links with any teaching assistants and/or communication support workers.
12. Support the teacher of the deaf's attempts to foster successful liaison.
13. Keep support staff informed of outcomes of home–school contact.
14. Alert support staff about parents' events and so on, and provide them with a calendar of relevant meetings.

Teacher of the deaf: _____

Key teacher: _____

Date: _____

Copies of this agreement circulated to: _____

_____

_____

_____

Glossary and abbreviations

Glossary

Aided thresholds – quietest sounds a person can hear when wearing hearing aids

Audiogram – chart recording the hearing of an individual

Audiometer – instrument used to determine hearing thresholds

Bilateral loss – bilateral hearing loss occurring in both ears

British Sign Language (BSL) – a visual–spatial language distinct from English, with its own vocabulary and grammar. Lip patterns, facial expression, body and head posture contribute to meaning.

Cochlear implant – microprocessor planted surgically on eighth auditory nerve

Conductive hearing loss – hearing loss due to the disturbance of any part of the mechanism that conducts sound into the inner ear

Congenital hearing loss – hearing loss due to genetic inheritance

Cued speech – a simple sound-based system devised to clarify the phonemes of spoken language, especially those that are ambiguous or invisible. It is a one-handed system with eight shapes using four positions near the mouth, used in conjunction with lip patterns.

Ear mould – plug shaped to fit an individual ear, through which acoustic output from a hearing aid is conveyed to the ear drum

Fingerspelling – an integral part of BSL using the fingers of both hands to represent the letters of the alphabet

Grommet – ventilation tube surgically inserted into ear drum

Lip reading / speech reading – a method of watching the face and lip patterns of a speaker in order to recognise different phonemes and groups of phonemes

Makaton vocabulary – structured selection of vocabulary taken from BSL, often used with children with severe learning difficulties. It helps the expression of essential needs

Otitis media – inflammation of the middle ear

Prosodic features – intonations, fluctuations in speech that enhance understanding/meaning

Receiver – pupil's part of the radio (FM) system

Recruitment – an unpleasant sensation experienced in certain cases of hearing loss, for example of cochlear origin. A sound is amplified through the hearing aid, causing unbearable loudness, pain and discomfort.

Residual hearing – hearing ability that remains in a case of severe or profound deafness

Sensori-neural loss – hearing loss that relates to the cochlea and/or auditory neural pathway, but not to the conductive mechanism of the ear

Signal to noise ratio – ratio of signal amplitude to noise amplitude in a particular situation

Sound Field System – system for amplifying a speaker's voice uniformly around a room

Speech reading – see *Lip reading*

Transmitter – teacher's part of radio FM system

Unilateral loss – unilateral hearing loss occurring in one ear only

For an explanation of the role of specific professions, see Chapter 8.

Abbreviations

APD – auditory processing disorder

BECTA – British Educational Communications and Technology Agency

BSA – British Society of Audiology

BSL – British Sign Language

CACDP – Council for the Advancement of Communication with Deaf People

CSW – community support worker

DDA – Disability Discrimination Act

DELTA – Deaf Education through Listening and Talking

DfES – Department for Education and Skills

DRC – Disability Rights Commission

LSA – learning support assistant

NDCS – National Deaf Children's Society

RNID – Royal National Institute for deaf and hard of hearing people

SCMO – Senior Clinical Medical Officer

SFS – Sound Field System

TA – teaching assistant

TC – Total Communication

ToD – teacher of the deaf

Resources

Note that publications that are not in print are available in libraries, and sometimes from the publisher.

References

DfES (2001), *Special Educational Needs Code of Practice*, Department for Education and Skills

Dillon, H. (2001), *Hearing Aids*, Boomerang Press

Flexer, C. (1994), *Facilitating Hearing and Listening in Young Children*, Singular Publishing

Maxwell, L.E. and Evans, G.W. (2000), 'The Effects of Noise on Pre-school Children's Pre-reading Skills', *Journal of Environmental Psychology*, 20, pp. 91–97

RNID (2004), *Effective Inclusion of Deaf Pupils into Mainstream Schools* (leaflet)

Further reading

BATOD (1994), *Guidelines for Teachers preparing Worksheets*, British Association of Teachers of the Deaf

DRC (2001), *Disability Discrimination Act: Code of Practice*, Disability Rights Commission

Gregory, S. and Hartley, G. (eds.) (1991), *Constructing Deafness*, Pinter / Open University

Groce, N.E. (1988), *Everyone here spoke Sign Language: Hereditary Deafness in Martha's Vineyard*, Harvard University Press

Lewis, S. (1998), 'Reading and Writing within an Oral/Aural Approach' in Gregory, S. *et al.* (eds.) *Issues in Deaf Education*, David Fulton

McCracken, W. and Laiode Kemp, S. (1997), *Audiology in Education*, Whurr Publishers

Maltby, M. Tate and Knight, P. (2000), *Audiology: An Introduction for Teachers and Other Professionals*, David Fulton

Martin, M. and Summers, I. (1999), *Dictionary of Hearing and Acoustics*, Whurr Publishers

NDCS (2004), *Deaf Friendly Nurseries and Pre-schools*, National Deaf Children's Society

NDCS (2004), *Deaf Friendly Schools*, National Deaf Children's Society

NDCS (2004), *Deaf Friendly Teaching*, National Deaf Children's Society

NDCS (2004), *Hearing Aids – A Guide*, National Deaf Children's Society

Powers, S. and Gregory, S. *et al.* (1999), *A Review of Good Practice in Deaf Education*, RNID for deaf and hard of hearing people (out of print)

RNID (2004), *Guidelines for Mainstream Teachers with Deaf Pupils in their Class*, RNID for deaf and hard of hearing people

RNID (2001), *Promoting Numeracy in Deaf People*, RNID for deaf and hard of hearing people

RNID (2001), *Using Residual Hearing Effectively*, RNID for deaf and hard of hearing people

Schuchman, J.S. (1999), *Hollywood Speaks: Deafness and the Film Entertainment Industry*, University of Illinois Press

Tryckeri, L. (2002), *Don't Limit your Senses – Sound and the Learning Environment*, Saint-Gobain Echophon

Webster, A. (1986), *Deafness, Development and Literacy*, Methuen

Both the RNID and the NDCS publish a wide range of useful literature, which is constantly updated. Full details of their publications can be found on the relevant websites.

Fiction, poetry and autobiography

Cookson, C. (2000), *Our John Willie*, G.K. Hall & Co.

Grant, B. (ed.) (1987), *The Quiet Ear: Deafness in Literature. An Anthology*, Andre Deutsch

Greenburg, J. (1983), *In this Sign*, Avon Books

Hughes, T. (1979), *Deaf School from Moortown*, Faber and Faber

Keller, H. (1963), *The Story of my Life*, Hodder and Stoughton

McCullars, C. (2001), *The Heart is a Lonely Hunter*, Penguin Books

Medoff, M. (1994), *Children of a Lesser God* (play), Dramatist's Play Service

Walker, L.A. (1987), *A Loss for Words*, Fontana Collins

Useful contacts

National Deaf Children's Society (NDCS)
15 Dufferin Street, London, EC1Y 8UR
020 7490 8656
Freephone helpline: 0808 800 8880

Royal National Institute for deaf
and hard of hearing people (RNID)
19–23 Featherstone Street, London, EC1Y 8SL
020 7296 8000
Freephone helpline: 0808 808 0123

British Association of Teachers of the Deaf (BATOD)
175 Dashwood Avenue, High Wycombe,
Buckinghamshire, HP12 3DB
secretary@batod.org.uk

British Deaf Association (BDA)
69 Wilson Street, London, EC2A 2BB
020 7588 3520

British Educational Communications
and Technology Agency (BECTA)
Millburn Hill Road, Science Park,
Coventry, CV4 7JJ
024 7641 6994

Council for the Advancement of Communication
with Deaf People (CACDP)
Durham University Science Park,
Block 4, Stockton Road, Durham, DH1 3UZ
0191 383 1155

Deaf Education through Listening and Talking (DELTA)
The Con Powell Centre, 3 Swan Court, Cygnet Park,
Peterborough, PE7 8GX
0845 1081437

Medical Research Council
Institute of Hearing Research Nottingham Clinical
Section, Eye Ear Nose and Throat Centre,
Queen's Medical Centre, Nottingham, NG7 2UH
0115 849 3351

Music and the Deaf
The Media Centre, 7 Northumberland Street,
Huddersfield, West Yorkshire, HD1 1RL
01484 483115

Useful websites

Ace Centre Advisory Trust: www.ace-centre.org.uk
(centre of information, support and training for
parents and professionals in the use of technology for
young people in education who have communication
difficulties, both in speaking and/or writing)

BATOD: www.batod.org.uk

BDA: www.signcommunity.org.uk

BECTA: www.becta.org.uk

CACDP: www.cacdp.org.uk

Cued Speech Association UK: www.cuedspeech.co.uk

DELTA: www.deafeducation.org.uk

Forest Books: www.Forestbooks.com
(supplies books, videos, DVDs and CD-Roms about
deafness, sign language and deaf issues)

Medical Research Council Institute of Hearing
Research: www.ihr.mrc.ac.uk

Music and the Deaf: www.matd.org.uk

National Deaf Children's Society: www.ndcs.org.uk

RNID: www.rnid.org.uk